LIFE
After Gastric Bypass

6 Steps to
Ensure Your
Weight Loss Success

**Katrina Segrave, RD, LDN, CSCS
and
Jerry Wayne,
Gastric Bypass patient success story**

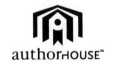

authorHOUSE™

1663 LIBERTY DRIVE, SUITE 200
BLOOMINGTON, INDIANA 47403
(800) 839-8640
WWW.AUTHORHOUSE.COM

First published by AuthorHouse 5/25/2006

ISBN: 1-4259-0378-9 (e)
ISBN: 1-4259-0377-0 (sc)

Printed in the United States of America
Bloomington, Indiana

This book is printed on acid-free paper.

Dedication

This book is dedicated to everyone affected by the disease of obesity. With love, it has been written specifically for those who have been riding the diet roller-coaster and battling their weight for years, often their entire lives.

It is our intention to send a life line to those who may be in the early stages of considering weight loss surgery. May the positive stories shared here give you the courage and inspiration to take the next step and schedule a consultation with an experienced bariatric program.

It is also our intent to send a ray of hope to those who have had gastric bypass and are fearful of returning hunger and the potential for weight re-gain.

May you find empowering information, inspiration and peace in the pages to come.

Katrina Segrave and Jerry Wayne

Acknowledgments

This book could not have come to fruition without the love and support of my *amazing* husband, Tom Segrave. Thank you, Tommy-boy, for believing in me. Thank you for being my best friend, my mentor and my biggest fan no matter what the current "Kat- project." I love you more and more every day and I love you *forever*.

A spiritual thanks to my Lord and Savior, Jesus Christ for the opportunity to touch so many lives in a positive way. After meeting with each and every patient I feel so humbled and grateful that I often bow my head in a prayer of thanks.

Heartfelt thanks to my co-author, Jerry Wayne. Your enthusiasm and commitment to writing this book is much the way you live your life – full on. Without you, I don't know if I would have ever put pen to paper and had this book to show for it. It's amazing how many people say, "I should write a book," but how many actually do it? Thanks to you we did it. You have such an amazing story to tell and so much love and positive energy to share with everyone around you. I loved you from the minute we met and I feel so blessed to have you and Rexanne in my life.

Special gratitude to:

Bobbie Lou Price, Dr. MacDonald and Dr. Chapman for the trust and confidence you bestow in me with each patient referral and speaking engagement. I appreciate and enjoy being a part of your esteemed medical care team.

Dr. Davidson, Dr. Classen and Donna Carter for your team-work and continued pursuit of medical excellence.

To each and every patient I have been blessed to work with over the years. You are my inspiration and my greatest teachers.

Together, Jerry and I offer special thanks to:

Ryan Segrave for your generous gift of time and editing expertise.

Mark Rosenberg of True Parallel Marketing for his creative talent and vision.

Janine Latus for her mentoring and encouragement.

Greg Lassiter of Champions Health and Fitness Center for his passion and dedication to his center members and the fitness industry. Thank you for letting us shoot our exercise photos at Champions.

Leslie Pepper, freelance writer and editor, for her brutal honesty and mentoring.

Johnny Wells of Ngage Design Studio for his excellence as a graphic artist.

Mary Ellen Wetherington of Ngage Design Studio for her web site design.

Tim Harper, freelance writer, author, and partner in Long Dash Publishing for his insight and editing expertise.

Jenn Handy of Author House for her professionalism and endurance which got us to the finish line.

Katrina Segrave and Jerry Wayne

And finally, to the love of my life, Rexanne! I thank you from the bottom of my heart for giving me total support on this project. From the day I came up with the crazy idea of writing a book and taking notes in a journal, to spending hours and hours on the phone or computer with Kat. I love you better than biscuits!

Kat, we did it! Let's celebrate! Nice shoes.

Jerry

CONTENTS

Foreword

Obesity is more than a condition or state of being. It is a disease that is running rampant in our country. A disease that has outpaced most other disease states. It affects millions of adults and children. The cost of obesity and it's associated conditions are staggering.

For the last decade I have been involved in the surgical management of obesity at the Brody School of Medicine at East Carolina University. Through the years, I have seen many patients positively change their lives with the help of gastric bypass surgery. The story you are about to read is one of our many success stories. Jerry Wayne chronicles his battle with obesity. He shares with us the trials and tribulations of being obese, multiple weight loss attempts, the workup for gastric bypass and his post-operative saga with hernias and plastic surgery. This is a very realistic, poignant and sometimes comical description of one man's experience with weight-loss surgery. Everyone's experience is unique, but I am sure that anyone who struggles with obesity, or who has undergone a gastric bypass will be able to relate to much of what is described in this story. Jerry is a true inspiration and a great advocate for obesity surgery. It has truly been my pleasure to have him as a patient.

William H. Chapman
Associate Professor of Surgery
Brody School of Medicine
East Carolina University

One

THE DAY I KNEW

As the adage goes, most people won't take action until their backs are up against the wall and there's nothing to do but come out swinging. Well, that's where I was.

It wasn't the fact that I had sleep apnea and needed a machine to keep me breathing at night. Nor was it the fact that I couldn't cross my legs, shop for clothes in regular stores, fit in a booth at a restaurant, or walk more than a few minutes without having to stop because of extreme back pain and shortness of breath. I, like many of you reading this book, had found ways to compensate for my physical limitations. And I was numb to all the jokes from kids and stares from adults. So, none of these things were a factor on what became "the day I knew."

The day I knew I had to do something – the day I knew I absolutely had to lose weight – was when I realized I had gotten so big that could not wipe my own backside. I couldn't get around my own massive belly or reach behind my own back to clean myself. It was an embarrassing secret I thought I would take to my grave. At that point I was well over 450 pounds.

When my wife, Rexanne, reads this book it will be the first she's ever heard about "the day I knew."

Contrary to popular belief, weight loss surgery is not the easy way out. It's a major life-altering choice that you and your family will have to live with for the rest of your lives. But now you have a life to live.

In the following chapters, I will tell my story – about a lifetime of obesity and how one decision changed my life. Then my friend and co-author, Katrina Segrave, will answer your nutrition and exercise questions and help you create your own personal program for success.

Katrina is an expert in her field and has shown me how to maximize my health and weight loss since my surgery. Today she inspires me to keep striving toward new levels of "my personal best," and we hope to share some of that inspiration with you in the pages to come.

Two

FROM WEIGHT WATCHERS TO ATKIN'S

Just like most of you, I've been on every diet in history. Not really, but sometimes it seems like it. Some of those diets even worked – for a while.

My dieting history dates back to grade school. My mom was trying her hardest to get me to slim down a little, but our neighbor wanted to me to be happy. Isn't it funny how we think food brings happiness? Sure, my mom would feed me, and feed me well. She just wanted me to cut down on the snacks and goodies between meals. So when I was hungry and probably shouldn't have been, I would walk over to Mrs. Garcia's house and plead my case. I wouldn't beg, exactly. But I must have been good at looking hungry. Certainly Mrs. Garcia seemed to think that my mom was trying to starve me into a svelte little boy. Of course Mrs. Garcia knew better, but it didn't matter. She would grab a loaf of bread, fix me a huge peanut butter and jelly sandwich, and give me a glass of milk to wash it down. She'd sit and watch me enjoy it and send me home.

Needless to say, my mom knew. She knew everything – everything except how to help me slim down.

My parents say there was a time in my childhood that I was actually skinny. I've even seen the pictures to prove it, but I sure don't remember. In fact I was big the day that I was born. "Aye, aye, aye, whatta bigga boy!" the doctor who delivered me shouted with his heavy Italian accent.

I'm told the nurses were taking bets on how much I weighed. I think they all underbid: Over 11 pounds and 23½ inches long.

"He's ready for a paper route," my dad marveled to my mother, who is only five-foot-three.

I really began to put on weight around fourth grade and to tell you the truth I don't care if I ever hear the word "husky" again. It was embedded in my brain growing up.

"He's not overweight, he's just husky for his age," the people who loved me said.

"He's a husky one isn't he?" polite strangers said. Those who weren't so polite said other things.

Then, of course, there were the words my mother used so often at Sears when shopping for school clothes. "Excuse me," she'd ask. "Where is your husky department?" I was one of the few kids who got his brothers' hand-me-down clothes early in life and then, as I got bigger, they got my hand-me-ups. I wish I'd bought stock in big and tall clothing stores back then.

My first major diet was Weight Watchers. I was in high school and weighed about 220 pounds, gaining more every year. So my mom and my Aunt Linda signed the three of us up for Weight Watchers. Every Wednesday evening we headed to a church in the town where I grew up in. Belleville, Michigan is a very small town and everyone knows one another, so it didn't take long for someone's mom who happened to be at the same Wednesday meetings to tell their son who they ran into at Weight Watchers.

But it didn't matter. I was there every week, a teenaged boy in a church full of women who all wanted me to succeed. I think some of them were more thrilled when I lost weight than when they did, including my Aunt Linda. She is one of the most motivated, strong-willed, independent and caring women I've ever known. She and my mom kept me motivated about losing weight and it worked for a while. I remember going back to that church for the first weigh-in and I had lost 10 pounds. We celebrated by going out to eat. Go figure.

Weight Watchers didn't last long. Two years later I was on my own and living in southwest Florida, working at my second gig in radio. The owners of the radio station were very into health and fitness, and they encouraged me to lose weight. They gave me a membership to a gym and even traded advertising to get me into the Physicians Weight Loss program. This program is based on a diet that consists of products sold through a doctor who gives you a weekly once-over. My first month was free thanks to the radio station. But my meager salary at the time didn't allow me to keep up with the program when I had to pay for it on my own.

Two radio jobs later I was back in Michigan and it was NutriSystem, with more products and more money and the same results: A little weight loss and less money in my pocket and more weight gained back after the program ended.

Then I was recruited by a hospital in Mt. Pleasant, Michigan to participate in a weight loss experiment called "The Diet That Lets You Cheat." There were 16 of us, all men, on a 2,000-calorie-a-day diet. Eight men were randomly chosen for the diet and exercise program and eight for the diet alone. I was on the diet program without exercise. It consisted of a strict diet of regular foods that changed every week for twelve weeks.

I will never forget the first day we weighed in at the hospital. They made us go into the basement and use the scales that they used to weigh laundry carts. I tipped the scales at 399 pounds. My first reaction was shame and embarrassment. I felt horrible. Then I was overjoyed, quietly and a bit guiltily, when other guys got on the scale and weighed even more than me.

Once a week we were allowed 300 free calories of what ever we wanted. I chose to use mine for three Miller Lites during Monday Night Football with the guys. The program was great and it really showed me how to change my eating habits.

We were taken to grocery stores and shown how to read labels to avoid the wrong or processed foods. We counted calories, measured foods, and we were even given lessons about choosing the best possible foods in the worst situations, such as restaurants, parties and holidays. I lost over 50 pounds in just six weeks on the program and 20 more when I was hospitalized with pneumonia.

I moved to North Carolina three weeks after being released from the hospital, and I kept the weight off for a while. But, without sounding like a total broken record, being new to the area and not knowing a soul, it became all too easy to wander off the diet and get back into my bad old drive-thru habits. Needless to say, the weight came back and then some.

After eight months in North Carolina I had gained some of the weight back. I also gained the love of my life. Obviously, I did try to watch my weight while in this wonderful relationship, but let's face it, I was still a big guy at about 340 pounds. Rexanne and I were married 15 months after we met. Soon the weight was creeping back up and before long I was back up to about 380 pounds.

Then the most significant invention in the history of mankind was introduced. Phen-Fen! That stuff was the greatest. Take two pills a day… never get hungry… watch the weight fall off. I was a new man. Once a month I would pay some wacky doctor a $40 office fee so he could take my blood pressure, weigh me and give me a 30-day prescription for Phen-Fen. This dude was my hero. I dropped 80 pounds in about four months and was under 300 pounds for the first time since high school. Rexanne was married to a new man. For Christmas my mother-in-law gave me my first pair of Lands' End jeans. I had a butt! It seemed for the first time in my adult life, I was going to be skinny. Nothing was going to stop me from being small.

Until Phen-Fen started killing people.

Three

GOD BLESS CARNIE WILSON

So this girl from the rock group Wilson Phillips decided to go public with her decision to have Gastric Bypass Surgery. Everyone knew who she was. The daughter of a Beach Boy, she sang with her sister and their friend Chynna Phillips. Wilson Phillips had some chart success in the 1990s and made several videos that each kept Carnie, who was far from slender, in the shadows. The spotlight focused on the other two women, who were both beautiful and slender. On tour, in videos, anywhere in public, Carnie was swathed in dark clothes designed to make her look a little slimmer. But hey, she could sing and she was the daughter of a Beach Boy.

Stomach stapling has been around for quite some time, but what Carnie announced she would do – Gastric Bypass, also called bariatric surgery – was new and different. Not to mention that the entire surgery was going to be on the Internet. Millions of people watching Carnie Wilson's stomach being stapled and stitched, then her intestines cut out and re-attached to her new stomach. I did not view the surgery, but I did read about it all over the Internet. I also kept up on her amazing weight loss success. I saw her on all of the news and talk shows. I saw her eat half of a grilled chicken salad on national television and tell the world that she was full. Full! Half of a grilled chicken salad would have just made me mad. But I was intrigued.

I started to look for doctors in North Carolina who performed the surgery. I didn't find as many as I had hoped. But there was a doctor in Durham who sent me oodles of information about himself, the surgery, and more about himself. I filled out an extremely lengthy question-naire about my life and my weight. It felt much like writing this book. The doctor wanted to know my diet history. Each and every diet I had ever been on, how many times I failed, and how much weight I gained back. There were questions about my family history and the sizes of my siblings. Not to mention the series of physiological questions and essays I had to write about why I thought I wanted this major surgery.

It didn't matter to me. It seemed to be a wonderful thing. Someone close to home performing the surgery at an unbelievable rate with great success. Or so I thought. After further investigation, I began to hear rumors about this doctor. Then suddenly he moved his practice out of Durham. Nobody knew why, but it didn't matter. He was not the guy for me.

My search for a doctor continued.

Four

SEEKING PROFESSIONAL HELP

I've worked in radio my entire adult life. For the last ten years I have been the program director at Oldies 107.9 WNCT in Eastern North Carolina. I started there in December 1994 and worked every morning from 5 a.m. until 10 a.m. on a show called "The Big Oldies Breakfast." Then I would use the rest of the day for producing commercials and programming the radio station.

I am proud to say that out of the ten years at Oldies 107.9 I have called in sick fewer than half a dozen times. I'm sure a few of those days were from a hangover and not due to an actual illness, but don't tell my boss. Sure, I would get sick, but I just worked through it and went home after the show. But one morning, when my alarm went off at the dreaded 4 o'clock, I was so sick and felt so badly that I had to have my wife call the guys at the station and tell them that I wouldn't be in. It was horrible. I had a fever and I ached all over, so I thought it was the flu. I stayed in bed the entire day and never got up except for the occasional fluids and to use the bathroom.

"We should get you to the doctor," Rexanne said.

"Nah," I said, typical man. "I'll be fine tomorrow."

Nope. The next morning I felt worse and called in sick again. When I was using the bathroom and what felt like pure fire came out of me instead of urine, I decided to call the doctor. Little did I know what this would mean for me.

My doctor, Dr. Goforth, is a great guy. He speaks to you like you are human, and not some alien from a planet far away. He is also very honest, and sometimes too honest. After running a few tests and some blood work, he announced, "You have a urinary tract infection."

Now I'm am far from a medical expert, but I was under the assumption that generally women were the unfortunate souls to get that affliction, which I now know as a U.T.I. Of course my initial response to this information from Dr. Goforth was, "How the hell did I get that?"

"I don't know, but we're going to find out," he responded.

It was at this point I wish I had kept my mouth shut. When he turned around from his medical cabinet it didn't take a brain surgeon to figure out what he was going to do with those rubber gloves and K.Y. jelly.

With the Dueling Banjos theme from the movie "Deliverance" ringing in my ears, I dropped my pants and tried to think about football. Dr. Goforth told me that he was checking my prostate, but if you ask me, I think he was rummaging around for hidden Christmas gifts. After he finished and handed me two Kleenex, I commented that the experience was little disturbing.

"Hey, Jerry," he said. "It wasn't exactly the highlight of my day, either."

The good news was that my prostate was fine. The bad news was that they still didn't know why I had the dreaded U.T.I. and they were going to send me to see a urologist named Dr. Cox. At that point I knew I was in trouble.

I was given some antibiotics that day, and I felt one hundred percent better. The medicine allowed me to go to work the next morning. Later that week I met with Dr. Cox. You have no idea the puns that were going through my mind while in the waiting room. Once I was called in, the nurse asked me a few questions, took my blood pressure, and told me to take off my clothes and put on the butt-baring gown. This last instruction I couldn't understand, but I did as I was told. Once the doc came in the room, put on rubber gloves and grabbed the K.Y. jelly, I knew.

Of course I had to ask why we were doing this again. Dr. Goforth assured me that my inner cave was fine. Dr. Cox told me that it was either up the cave or he could send a probe down my shaft – a much smaller hole. So after more ESPN highlights going through my head and digging for gold, I was given the complementary Kleenex.

"OK Jerry, you can get dressed and I'll be back in a minute," he said.

As it turns out, the doctors never did figure out why I had the U.T.I. They believe it was just a fluke.

This infection probably wasn't a turning point in my health decline, but it was the point that sticks out in my mind. The weight was taking its toll on me in more ways than one. My back started hurting first, and it was sore constantly. Walking for more than just a few minutes would produce a pain my back that I would not wish on my worst enemy. Then it was my knee. Just getting in and out of the car was a chore. There was always a dull pain to daily remind me of my size. It was the loss of breath that was really getting to me. Just getting out of a golf cart and walking to my golf ball during games would cause me to huff and puff.

That's when I decided to sit down with Dr. Goforth and really consider this gastric bypass thing I had been investigating on the Internet. We talked about all of the diets that I've been on in the past and their ultimate failures. He explained to me that I was slowly killing myself and the only thing going for me was age. He knew the problems associated with obesity were catching up with me, and he did a wonderful job of explaining what was coming. Diabetes, heart attacks, stroke, and ultimately an early death were on his list. To this day I don't know if he was trying to scare the fat off me, but it worked. That was the day that I decided to go through with the most drastic decision in my life.

The next question out of Dr. Goforth's mouth was, "Where do you want to have the surgery?" I had no idea. We talked about the breakthroughs in gastric bypass surgery, and the number of hospitals that were performing the surgery. We decided on Duke University Hospital in Durham, N.C. The next day he typed a letter summarizing my situation and recommending me for the surgery and sent it off to the powers that be. It wasn't long before I was knee deep in the beginning of my new life.

Five

OFF TO DUKE

Now that I had a hospital, it was time to "qualify" for the surgery. I began a series of tests that were necessary before we could submit a proposal to my insurance company. Heck, I thought if you were so overweight the hospital would clear you for the surgery if you could afford it, or if your insurance company would cover you. Luckily, most tests were done locally so I didn't have to drive the nearly 100 miles to Durham for all of them.

As my doctor began scheduling a series of tests required by the hospital, I attacked the paperwork. I received a huge packet of information and forms in the mail. I remember giving my history of being fat. The forms were to give the doctors all of the diets I had been on in my lifetime. They wanted to know all of my ailments. I had plenty, so it took a while to fill in the forms.

Rexanne and I went through form after form giving them everything they asked for, including several paragraphs of why I wanted to have gastric bypass surgery. At first I didn't know what to say. But once I got started, the words flowed like a raging river. I talked about how I longed to be able to do things like a normal person. I know what you're thinking, "Who is normal these days?" To me, normal was anything other than being fat. I wanted to do normal things. Things that skinny people take for granted everyday.

Like bending over to tie my shoes so that the knot wasn't cocked to one side of the shoe, because I had to throw my foot over my knee and tie it from the side.

Like buying clothes while on vacation.

Never worrying about sitting in a folding chair. Picking up loose change off the floor without bending my whole body in half, with one leg in the air like a ballerina, then bouncing down until I could grab one coin at a time.

Going through a turnstile by walking straight through without turning to the side and standing on my tiptoes so my belly would go over the top.

Not wearing a T-shirt every time I went swimming.

Having a waist to hold up my pants, instead of huge belts cinched as tight as possible to keep them from falling to my ankles.

Running.

Crossing my legs (now one of my favorite things to do).

Never having strangers stare at me.

Riding a roller coaster.

Sitting in a booth in a restaurant instead of a table.

Being able to look straight down and see my shoes.

Walking for more than five minutes without being out of breath.

Swinging a golf club... the right way.

But the one thing that embarrassed me the most – I'm sure skinny people take this for granted – was asking the flight attendant for a seat-belt extension.

The hospital staff did not have to read much to know why I wanted this surgery, and that I was committed. But they still wanted a lot from me, and I gave them everything they wanted – including blood.

My physical tests were completed at Lenoir Memorial Hospital in Kinston, N.C. The usual series of blood work was drawn for just about everything you can think of. Then it was a standard stress test to find out how my ticker was. Luckily, my heart was pumping just fine, even though I thought I was going to die on that treadmill. The stress test led to some type of respiratory test. I saw a specialist who put me in a small cylinder to perform various breathing tests. After about an hour of huffing and puffing, this dude makes the rocket-science statement of the decade to an over-400-pound man.

"It appears your extra weight causes you to lose your breath easily," he said.

Duh!

Everything they check you for weighs heavily on the insurance company's decision to cover your surgery or not. So after every test result comes back you find yourself preparing for bad news. Or, rather, two waves of bad news. First, if they find something you didn't know you had, that's depressing. Second, the new diagnosis might mean you have to put off the Gastric Bypass Surgery.

I was pleased when an ultrasound showed I didn't have gallstones. I thought that meant that I could have laproscopic surgery – small incisions – rather than the "open" procedure that starts with the surgeon cutting you from chin to belly button. But it didn't matter in the end. I found out that at my size having the laproscopic surgery was not an option.

As it turned out, I was a pretty healthy fat man. Mostly because of my age, just a little over thirty years old, the complications of obesity hadn't really started affecting me yet. But the health issues weren't far off, and the folks at Duke UMC and my insurance company knew it. So I was accepted for the surgery and the insurance process began.

I remember the day Rexanne and I headed to Duke University Hospital in Durham for a meeting with the doctors and nurses in the bariatric department. During the drive we talked about the surgery and tried to plan our lives around my new life. It was really more small talk than anything, because I was scared to death and didn't feel like holding a deep conversation. Later Rexanne told me, "I was as scared as you were."

When we arrived at the hospital I was given more forms to fill out as we waited in a room with many other people who obviously were there for the same reason. I didn't know it was going to be a group session. Actually we were divided into a couple of groups and taken into two different conference rooms. The doctors and nurses took turns talking to each room. The doctor who visited with us first explained exactly how the surgery would be performed, depending on which procedure we were having, and what to expect after the surgery. He took questions from patients and a couple of nurses explained what still needed to be done before the surgery and how we should prepare for the big day. We spoke with other office staffers about insurance and then broke up into individual rooms for a doctor's checkup.

That's when things started going downhill. Just as I was called back to the examination room, a young woman in a white coat told me to see her regarding insurance after I saw the doctor. Crap! I knew it was way too early for an approval, so I was a little nervous.

Once we were in the examination room I went through pretty routine stuff: blood pressure, pulse, listening to my heart and lungs, etc. Then I was hooked up to a machine with all of these wires and it spit out a total body analysis. It gave the doctor my total body fat, amount of muscle tissue, and water weight. Then came the first bad news of the day. The doctor told me that at almost 450 pounds I would be one of the biggest patients they would have ever performed the surgery on. The hospital would have to order a special bed for me to support my weight in the operating room. Ironically, that bed would have to come from Pitt County Memorial Hospital in Greenville. My radio station is just one mile from that hospital. The doctor explained to me that the East Carolina Brody School of Medicine was located there, and that they were the cutting edge for this surgery. In fact, they had all been trained and consulted by Dr. Pories, a man known globally for his breakthroughs with the Rou-en-Y procedure, the method used in bariatric surgery. At that point, the question was not only on my mind, but Rexanne's and the doctor's as well.

Why was I not having this surgery in Greenville?

At the end of my examination the doctor wanted me to schedule a sleep study to test me for sleep apnea, and suggested I find a place closer to home. I thought that would be my final hurdle on the road to my new life. I was wrong. On the way out of the hospital, as requested, I stopped by the desk of the lady working on the insurance forms. She told us that if I were approved for the surgery, my insurance would only pay for half of the expense; my insurer did not participate in a plan with

Duke. The surgery cost back then was close to $30,000. Half was not an option. The words from that woman's mouth still ring in my ears, "Why don't you call Pitt Memorial Hospital in Greenville? They accept your insurance, and they have a pretty good bariatric surgery department."

Back to the drawing board.

Six

DYING FOR A GOOD NIGHT'S SLEEP

After the Duke visit, I scheduled the sleep study near the new hospital of choice, Pitt County Memorial in Greenville, N.C. I began the entire process over again. Fortunately, I, along with the great staff of Oldies 107.9, have raised a great deal of money for their Children's Hospital. By the time this book is in print, the total will be well over $1 million, so it wasn't too hard to make a few calls and get in contact with the powers that be. That's when I discovered that there was a waiting list of more than three hundred people, and it would be more than a year before I could have the surgery. I was tempted to give up right then, but I didn't. Instead I scheduled a preliminary meeting with a surgery staff nurse for the next week.

The meeting was much like my one and only meeting at Duke, just with fewer people. I waited in a small room with other folks who were obviously there for the same reason. We were given details on the entire surgical process. Everything was almost the same as what Duke presented, which didn't surprise me since this staff had trained many of the people at Duke. The biggest difference was that this was the very beginning for everyone in that room but me. They knew nothing about the surgery, and it was pretty amazing to watch their reaction to how many hoops they would have to jump through before becoming a candidate.

I was all smiles because I had been jumping through those very same hoops for months. I just prayed I wouldn't have to do it all again. Near the end of the meeting, as we were individually taken into a small examination room to meet with the doctor, the nurse we were meeting with asked us if we had any more questions. I saw this as an opportunity to start telling as many people as possible that I had already been down this road, and start finding out how I could fast-track my way to surgery. She asked me what had been done up to that point for surgery preparation. I told to her about the trip to Duke, and about all the tests that were complete except for the sleep study, which already had been scheduled for the next week.

She agreed that I was well ahead of the other folks in the room. Insurance would be the biggest remaining issue, but the sleep study would help speed along the process, she said, because I was almost sure to be diagnosed with "sleep apnea."

"What makes you think I probably have sleep apnea?" I asked the nurse.

She said she had noticed that I dozed off three or four times during the group meeting. "Do you nod off a lot during the day?" she inquired.

"I get sleepy every now and then in the afternoon," I told her. "But I get up at four o'clock every morning." I was lying. The truth is, I was falling asleep several times throughout the day, and it didn't matter if was morning, midday, or afternoon. In fact, I can't count how many times I had fallen asleep while driving in the middle of the day. Luckily I had always started back awake before having a serious accident.

I wasn't entirely sure what sleep apnea was, but I quickly educated myself. Sleep apnea, which is caused by the relaxation of the tissue of the soft palate, deep in the throat, blocks your airways and causes you to stop breathing at night. Overweight people are particularly susceptible. Without air, your body wakes you up several times throughout the night in order to keep you from suffocating. This ultimately means a sleepless night, or at best a night with episodic, restless sleep rather than the kind of deep sleep that restores your body and spirit. In some severe cases, people have died in their sleep because of sleep apnea. In many more cases where undiagnosed sleep apnea is mistaken for no more than loud and frequent snoring, grumpy spouses have taken their pillow to the spare room or the couch to get away from their lumberjack of the night.

On the evening I arrived at the sleep center, I had followed all the instructions. I had no alcohol for the previous twenty-four hours, no caffeine after noon of that day and no naps. I had been told to wear whatever I would normally wear to bed at night, and to bring an overnight bag with a change of clothes for the next morning. I thought about telling them that I slept in the nude, until the staff told me about the video cameras and the dozens of wires that would be attached to me. They showed me my room. It looked much like a hotel room even though they really did try to give it a homey feel. But, with the camera in the top corner of the room and a monitor system above the headboard, I knew this was not going to be a good night's sleep.

They asked me to go ahead and change into my sleeping attire, then meet them in their monitoring area were they would prep me for the sleep study. Between the numerous wires, and the glue they used to attach them on my head and body, I started to feel like Frankenstein. I was wired up better than a home theater system. They plugged me into the wall next to the bed. I was instructed to get into bed, try to get comfortable, watch a little TV and get a good night's sleep.

The first time a voice came from the little speaker above the bed, it was about midnight. The voice instructed me to avoid sleeping on my side because it interfered with the tangled web of wires hanging from my skull. The sensors couldn't get a good reading. So much for the getting comfortable part of this sleep study. At about 1 a.m. I heard the same friendly voice from the mini-speaker; this time they were letting me know that someone was coming into the room to hook me up to yet another machine. A guy came in, and reached for a hose attached to the wall with a Darth Vader-like mask on the end of it. Even though I did not need an explanation for what he was going to do with the mask, I did want to know how it worked and what to expect. As soon as he spoke, I knew right away he was the voice from the speaker. He explained that the mask and hose were attached to an adjustable machine; he called it a "C-PAP," on the other side of the wall. He said the mask would fit over my nose and he would adjust the straps so that it was snug but comfortable. It was anything but comfortable.

In a quick non-professional description, the C-PAP machine is designed to assist sleep apnea sufferers with breathing while they sleep. It is a little machine that sits on the nightstand next to the bed along with a long hose that is attached to the machine at one end. On the other end is the triangular mask that really resembles a mask a fighter pilot might wear. The mask fits over your nose and is held on with adjustable straps that fit over your head. The machine pumps air continuously into your lungs through your nose, keeping your airways open and your oxygen level up.

Once the mask was on my nose and the straps adjusted over and around the dozens of wires, the man from the speaker started asking me some yes or no questions. My answers had to be short because if I opened my mouth, a blast of air shot out instead of my voice. At that point I was getting a little frustrated. The man from the speaker, now standing next to me, asked if the mask was too tight or too loose.

"Can you breathe all right?" he wondered. "Just breathe deeply through your nose. You'll sleep better than you have in years."

It sounded good in theory, but in reality things didn't get any better. I did fall asleep pretty quickly, probably because it was early in the morning and I was beat, but it didn't last long. The minute I turned in my sleep, the mask slipped out of position. Air started leaking out from the side, making a noise like someone letting air out of a balloon a little at a time. It was annoying and I became more irritated. After several failed attempts to fix it myself, I had to call for assistance from the voice. He reappeared promptly and pleasantly, and began to work on my mask by readjusting and tightening until I was ready for dreamland again. It was more like a nightmare.

Over the course of the next hour or so we not only went through several readjustments, we went through a couple of different masks, and my blood pressure went through the roof. I'm not one to lash out at someone just doing his or her job, but at 3 a.m. and with hardly any sleep, anything goes. After a little temper tantrum that scared the attendant into calling for reinforcements, things became even more interesting.

The woman who came in was obviously in charge of the staff, and just a few words away from being in charge of me. She ordered everyone out of the room and pulled up a chair to sit next to me. I was already on the side of the bed. She explained to me, in a calm but forceful voice, that I had not been asleep for a long enough period of time to take an accurate reading for the doctors. I needed to be asleep for at least two continuous hours and if I didn't calm down and cooperate, they would make me come back again for a full night's test. She then gave me the choice – go home and come back again another night or give it one last shot.

"One more shot," I said.

She seemed pleased and promised to try something else that she thought would work. She wanted me to complete the test, too.

She opened up the door called out a few orders to the folks in the monitoring room. Before I knew it, there were four people in my room working on me like a NASCAR pit crew. They unplugged my hose from the wall, brought in a machine about the size of a small duffle bag, and placed it on the nightstand. They reattached my hose to it and attached another new, slightly bigger mask to the other end of the hose. She then ordered them all out of the room again and began to adjust the mask onto my face and head, making sure it was snug but not too tight. She told me to lie on my back, get as comfortable as I could, and breath deeply though my nose. I didn't have a choice. The amount of force coming from the mask was unbelievable; my chest rose and fell with every breath as I closed my eyes and concentrated on my breathing.

When she came into my room one last time, it was to wake me up. I had been asleep for more than two hours and I felt like it had been a solid night's sleep. She congratulated me on being a great patient; she was lying, but I appreciated her help in getting me through the test. "We got what we need to complete the study," she concluded. "The doctor will go over the results with you next week."

I was untangled from the wires and glue, and allowed to shower and dress. The staff gave me an appointment to meet with the doctor, and I was at work by 6 a.m. and ready for the show.

It took three days to wash off all of the glue.

Seven

BLOWN AWAY

The next week I was back at the sleep center, in the daytime, to meet with Dr. Lee, a tiny little man with glasses. He was full of energy, bouncing around the examination room while he explained the results of the sleep study.

"Jerry Wayne, you stopped breathing so much we thought we would have to shock you," he said as he held his hands in the air like he was using the paddles of a defibrillator.   He then opened my chart and showed me my sleep pattern. I didn't understand much of it until he said, "You stop breathing hundreds of times a night. You get no oxygen! You could die!" That I understood.

Bottom line, my obesity was causing my airway to close off more than four hundred times every night, sometimes for up to a minute or more. That was the reason I was waking up several times during the night to use the bathroom. The lack of deep sleep was the reason I was tired all day long, and why I fell asleep at my desk and even while driving. But there was a solution.

Dr. Lee explained that on the night of the sleep study, the staff at first constantly increased the airflow to the C-PAP machine. When the C-PAP was at its maximum and I still stopped breathing, they brought in the bigger machine, called a BI-PAP, and put it on the nightstand. The BI-PAP kicks up the airflow to a whole new level.

I still almost maxed that machine out, but it helped me sleep and not wake up every couple of minutes. Dr. Lee showed my levels on the chart after they had hooked me up to the BI-PAP machine. There was a tremendous difference. I never stopped breathing and got more good healthy sleep in those two short hours than I had over the course of a week. I was going to need a BI-PAP at home. Before I left the sleep center, we went through one more training session on how to use and properly care for the BI-PAP machine. Then they set an appointment with a home medical supply company to bring the machine to my house for yet another training session and fitting.

It's amazing to me how total strangers got excited about the fact I was going to depend on a breathing apparatus for the rest of my life. Maybe it's because the folks at the sleep center consider it another victory in the fight against sleep apnea, and the folks at the home medical supply store now have one more monthly income from the insurance company and me. Whatever the reason, they were happy.

I, on the other hand, was not especially euphoric. I had to go home and explain to my wife that I frequently stopped breathing at night with the possibility of dying and we were going to have a strange bedfellow. Don't get me wrong. Rexanne was very supportive about my health; she would allow supermodels to give me mouth-to-mouth all night if that's what it took. But it was still a humbling experience. Once that mask goes on there is no cuddling, no second goodnight kiss or even pillow talk. In fact, between the noise of a small air compressor – and enough pressure going through my nose that if I opened my mouth the sheets would blow off the bed – there wasn't any talking at all. Rexanne and I still joke about that. All in all, Rexanne was fantastic about the entire experience and swears that it never bothered her. She said anything was better than my God-awful snoring

Eight

FINAL HURDLE...INSURANCE

We've all got to have insurance. We hate to pay for it, but we sure are glad it's there when we need it. Everyone has an insurance story and most are horror stories. But trying to convince an insurance company that you are a qualified candidate for bariatric surgery just plain stinks.

It's not just hoops they want you to jump through, it's hoops twenty feet high, set on fire, on the edge of a cliff with dozens of insurance people around hoping you don't make it through. OK, maybe it's not that bad, but it sure feels like it. Let's face it, the surgery is not cheap and it shouldn't be. If it were inexpensive, every person on the planet looking to lose thirty pounds would sign up.

By the time my sleep apnea was diagnosed, all of the tests and doctors' appointments were beginning to pay off. The hospital staff in Greenville kept in touch with the insurance company and gave them all the test results from the past few months – including the sleep study that determined I would be using an expensive machine for the rest of my life if I didn't have the surgery. It didn't take the insurance company long to deliberate my case, and I was approved for the surgery.

Once final approval came from my insurance company, it was time to get a surgery date and meet with the anesthesiologist. We listened intently as the anesthesiologist gave us the complete details of what to expect during surgery and discussed any possible risks and complications.

He explained a breathing tube would be inserted during surgery and if I weren't breathing well enough on my own following surgery, he would have to reinsert it. I wish I'd paid more attention to that part.

By the end of that week – it was late July – I received the call I'd been waiting for: a surgery date. The process that began in November of the previous year was about to have a date. I was so nervous my hands were shaking and it was hard to write. The staff wanted to schedule me for Friday, August 30th, just a little more than a month away. When I hung up the phone I felt like I was going to be sick. Then I called Rexanne and reality set in.

I had a surgery date. I was going to have an operation that would change my life forever – one way or another, successful or not. Rexanne and I were on the phone with each other but we didn't say much. By the time we met at home that night we realized there was a great deal of planning involved before surgery. We had just about a month to get our ducks in a row, or so we thought. The next day the hospital called again to tell me there was a cancellation. Would I be willing to move my surgery to August 9th, less than two weeks away? I said "yes," then called Rexanne and we both freaked out.

Nine

FAT SATURDAY!

The weekend before my surgery, Rexanne and I invited our friends to the beach for a "Fat Saturday Party." Similar to Fat Tuesday, it was a bunch of friends eating, drinking, and being very merry. It was my last chance to really let loose and enjoy myself before surgery and we wanted all of our friends to be a part of it. Everyone was encouraged to bring an appetizer or a dessert to share. I cooked a huge shrimp boil filled with potatoes, corn, sausage, and plenty of shrimp.

There were many great people at the party, and we ate, drank, talked, and danced until the wee hours of the morning. It was a fantastic night I will never forget even though I partied hard. But times have changed since then; everybody who was there can now eat and drink me under the table.

Ten

FOUR OUNCES TO FREEDOM

A few days before my surgery, I met with Dr. Chapman, who would perform the operation. He explained the Roux-en-Y procedure again, and what to expect after. Since I was too big for the laproscopic procedure, I would have an open surgery with an incision that started just above my belly button and went about eight inches toward my chest.

The healing time with an open procedure is longer and there is greater risk for infection and hernia, but the operation itself was the same. Dr. Chapman drew a rough illustration showing how he would remove part of my intestine, re-attach it with a smaller opening from my new, smaller stomach that would be the size of an egg and hold about four ounces of food. I went home thinking about how much four ounces actually is. After just a few minutes of research on the Internet I discovered that four ounces is exactly one half cup, eight tablespoons, about six strawberries, one kiwi fruit, two shots of liquor, twenty-five mini pretzels, six slices of cheese. And as my buddy Steve Kornegay says, "Four ounces is just one good martini."

After Dr. Chapman and I met, I had to sign more paperwork than I did the first time I bought a house. The hospital staffer with the paperwork gave me a little brown bag with a list of instructions and special soap to use the night before and the morning of surgery. A nurse told me to have only have caffeine- free, clear liquids twenty-four hours before surgery and nothing after midnight.

My parents arrived, with my niece Samantha, the Wednesday before my surgery. I took Friday off so we could spend the day at our "place at the beach." They had never been to Atlantic Beach and I wanted to show them the little piece of heaven Rexanne and I call the "tin-a-minium, " much like a condominium except it has wheels. All right, it's a mobile home, fourteen feet wide and seventy feet long.

It was not an extremely hot day in August by North Carolina standards – only in the middle eighties instead of the normal mid-nineties – but to my family from Michigan, it was hot! My dad loved it and the minute we hit the beach he removed his shirt, something I hadn't done in years, so he could soak up the sun and enjoy the white sandy beach and the sound of the ocean.

My mom, on the other hand, looked like a wet sponge, sweating profusely within seconds of being under the blazing sun. This is a trait she had passed on to me, since up until that point in my life I wore shorts just about year round because I was always hot. It took only a few minutes for mom to use all the tissues she had in her purse to wipe the sweat off her face before she asked us if we were ready to go. Of course dad said no, but he didn't win that argument.

We headed back to the "Redneck Riviera," another term of endearment for our trailer at the beach. Mom and Samantha stayed indoors and cooled off while dad and I sat in Adirondack chairs, enjoying a beer and each other's company. Soon we headed to historic Beaufort for some shopping and some lunch at Clawson's, a great little restaurant Rexanne and I have been going to for years. It really was a great way to relax and try not to think about the surgery the next day.

But the surgery was on everyone's mind. We all tried to shut out thoughts about all the many things that can go wrong, especially in this kind of major operation. The drive home from the beach was quiet. My Mom had already asked me every question possible about the surgery. I'm not sure I gave her the correct answers, but I did answer everything she asked. The silence was fine with me. My mind was about twenty-four hours away.

That night Rexanne and I took Mom, Dad and Samantha to a little restaurant called Ribeye's, great steaks, a wonderful salad bar, and just one minute from the house. Perfect. I will never forget how guilty my

Mom felt about eating in front of me as I could only have clear liquids. It was a long night.

The next morning I showered with the special soap that the hospital provided, and packed my overnight bag with toiletries and clothes for the trip home. My surgery was scheduled bright and early so Rexanne and I had to be at the hospital by 6 a.m., which was fairly easy for both of us since we didn't get much sleep. My parents would arrive at the hospital later that morning. The drive to Greenville from Snow Hill takes only twenty minutes and it is a daily commute for me at 5 each morning, but there was something different about that morning. Normally I'm in a hurry, pushing the speed limit, following my daily routine and keeping an eye on the clock so I arrive at the same time everyday. Not that day.

We left a little later than my normal routine, about 5:30 a.m. My senses were heightened, and things seemed to be moving almost in slow motion. I remember how humid it was; the sun was already piercing the treetops. If I broke the speed limit, it couldn't have been by more than a few miles per hour. I remember paying closer attention to the surroundings of the road, seeing things that I had never noticed before. Which houses had lights on inside and out, a woman arriving at the gas station to open up, and wondering what river the guys in the truck pulling the bass boat were going to be fishing in. Rexanne and I talked, but not about anything important. We held hands and in between awkward moments of silence I pointed out places along the road that I would normally spot deer on my way to work. I talked and drove; she listened and rode.

When we arrived at Pitt Memorial Hospital, I parked in the pay lot and we went in the main entrance. The woman at the front desk gave me a little paging device that buzzed and lighted up when it was our turn to go in. At that point I wasn't nervous. I even went to get a newspaper out of the box to keep us occupied during the wait. When I got back to our seats I asked Rexanne what section of the paper she would like to read, we realized it was the previous day's paper. Just as we started to chuckle together the pager went off, and we both jumped. The nervousness hit me like a lead pipe and I felt nauseated.

When Rexanne and I reported to the front desk, they did not take my pager as I expected. Instead we were directed down the hall to the surgical waiting room. We waited for the pager to go off again. It wasn't long. I walked down the hall and gave my name to the nurse. She walked us back to a room that had several beds with a curtain pulled around each. She pointed to the giant heavy-duty bed that was reserved for me, and instructed me to take off my clothes and get into one of those hospital gowns that doesn't cover your butt. She told Rexanne to put all of my clothes into a plastic bag; she could bring it to my room later. Rexanne was then asked to step out of the room so they could make preparations for surgery.

It was less than five minutes later that an orderly came through the curtain wheeling a rolling cart with towels, a bowl of water, shaving cream, and a razor. He introduced himself and explained he needed to shave my enormous stomach where the doctors were going to make their incision. After a few moments he was done and gave me a wet washcloth and towel to clean up and dry off.

After he left I heard some familiar voices and knew right away who was there. Rexanne came through the curtain again, this time with my parents and Claire, the preacher from our church, whom I had nicknamed our "Cool Chick Preacher." There was little small talk between one another and then Claire led us all in prayer. After the prayer Claire wished me luck and excused herself and left me with my parents and Rexanne so we could talk before they wheeled me back to the surgical prep area.

First my Mom and Dad gave me best wishes and assured me they would be right there when I woke up. Then they left Rexanne and I alone so we could have some privacy. Of course I tried to make light of the situation, even though I could see how frightened Rexanne was. I made my usual jokes and held her hand and never once thought I wouldn't see her again. Even minutes away from having my stomach cut wide open, I never fully grasped the concept that some people did die from this surgery. Not many, but some. An orderly showed up to wheel me and my bed to the operating theater. I kissed Rexanne and told her how much I loved her.

"Hey," I demanded of the orderly. "Does this big ol' bed have four-wheel-drive? If it don't you might need a hand to get it moving." He laughed and got me rolling with no problem. Rexanne laughed, too, and it was a good last sound to hear as I headed down the hallway. In my adult life I have never had surgery. I had tubes put in my ears well over twenty years ago but I don't remember much about it. So as my bed rolled down the hallway I thought about how strange it seemed to be paraded past everyone. Hospital employees, visitors, anyone in the hall could see this whale of man being wheeled away on a vast portable bed. As I watched the fluorescent lights and ceiling tiles slide by above me, I thought to myself, "All of the technology and brilliance in this huge hospital, and no one considered building a private hall to the pre-op room."

When we arrived in the holding room the orderly parked me next to another man. By the size of him, he was probably having the same surgery. A nurse came over and went to work on me. She introduced herself as she started to put in an I.V. and hooked me up to a monitor. By then other nurses came over after they recognized me. They made a little fuss over me, talked about the radio station, and joked about some of the wackier things I've done over years on the morning show.

After a few minutes they went back to their duties and my nurse told me it wouldn't be long before someone would give me drugs to relax me a bit before surgery. That short while turned into about an hour, and I was starting to get really uncomfortable. When you are four hundred fifty pounds, not many beds are comfortable, especially a hospital bed. So the nurse gave me something to make me relax and the next thing I knew my anesthesiologist was waking me up.

"Sorry," he said. "Things are a little behind schedule. It's still going to be a while before we take you into the O.R." He told me it was just about lunchtime, which was about three hours past my scheduled surgery time. He assured me he would be back to give me something to calm my nerves right before surgery. I was still loopy from whatever the nurse had given me earlier and I wondered what he had that the nurse didn't.

A few minutes later I noticed that the other large fellow wasn't next to me any more. They must have taken him in already. I asked my nurse about him and she confirmed my guess.

"You're next," she said. I dozed off again.

The next time I woke up, it was because of a minor commotion around my bed. The nurse and the orderly were getting ready to move me into the operating room. Suddenly I was wide awake, and all of the nerves were back. "Where's that dude with the good drugs?" I wondered.

By the time they had the bed ready to travel, the anesthesiologist arrived in full scrubs, a cap, booties over his shoes, and a mask pulled down around his neck. He brandished a hypodermic needle. "We're ready for you in the O.R.," he said, then injected something he called Versed into my I.V. "See you in a few minutes."

Instantly I had a funny feeling as the drug entered my veins. It seemed like my entire body was going limp as they began to wheel me though the public hallway again. I don't remember entering the operating room and I only vaguely remember the surgical team asking me to slide from the bed onto the operating table. My thoughts were a little clearer as my naked backside hit the cold stainless steel of the operating table. I wondered why they were stretching both of my arms straight out from my body on extensions that came out from the table. My fat was hanging over the edges. The anesthesiologist told me he was giving me another injection and I would wake up in the recovery room a few hours later. That was the last thing I remember.

Eleven

A DISC JOCKEY WHO CAN'T SPEAK!

When I woke up the first thing I saw was my mother. The next thing I saw was a white tube coming from my throat.

"It's a breathing tube," Mom explained, gently. "Don't try to talk."

She told me that the surgery went fine, but when they removed the breathing tube after surgery, I had trouble breathing on my own. She also told me I was in the recovery room.

My mom must have been able to tell by the look in my eyes that I wanted to know where Rexanne was. She said the surgery had gone well into the afternoon and Rexanne finally left with our friends George and Lisa Ritko to get a bite to eat. She had been at the hospital all day without a break and they told her I would be out for quite a while.

Mom talked to me about the day and how long it had been. My friends had stopped by to check on me throughout the day and my buddy Brent Bennett, who sings with a group called the "Carolina Beach Club," didn't leave the hospital until he knew I was OK.

A nurse entered to check my vital signs and told me I had a device near my hand with a button to push if I was in pain. "That will release morphine into your veins," she said. I pushed it, it beeped, and I felt a warm sensation in my arm as I fell asleep again.

Even though I had been in and out of consciousness, I remember the first time Rexanne walked into the recovery room. I gave her the biggest smile possible with a tube down my throat, and she smiled back. Till this day she swears I was smiling with my eyes. From that moment on she never left my side.

Later that evening I moved to the intensive care unit because I still had the breathing tube that needed constant monitoring. Rexanne made it clear that she was not leaving my room, so the nurses in the ICU moved in a cot for her.

Whenever I woke up during the night – which was quite often – I looked over to see if Rexanne was still there. She was.

The next morning when we were both awake, I wanted to communicate. I made a writing motion with my hand and someone brought in a pad and pen. I wrote Rexanne little notes all day. My Mom and Dad were the first visitors, but only for a few minutes. They talked and I listened, reassured. They promised to be back soon.

I remember while they were gone I kept asking Rexanne what time it was by pointing to my wrist. After about the fourth time in five minutes, she was curious. "Why is it so important for you to know exactly what time it is?" she asked.

I jotted down that there were about eight minutes in between the allotted morphine drips, and I was eager for the next jolt of juice. She laughed the way only Rexanne can when she knows that I am up to something.

During the next ICU visitation period my parents arrived along with my buddy Chris Parham. He is one of my best friends, and works as the golf course superintendent at Greenville Country Club. Just like everyone who came to visit, he talked and I listened. Then I motioned to the hat that he had on his head. "It's the new G.C.C. hat," he said. "You like it? OK, buddy, I'll get you one." And he did.

I'm not sure what time that first full day in recovery they decided to take the breathing tube out, but I was not going to argue. "You still shouldn't try to talk," the nurse said.

Yeah, right, I thought, just try and keep a disc jockey from talking after nearly twenty-four hours of enforced silence. She said that while they were removing the tube, I should try to cough and not stop. Then she signaled to me with a nod to start coughing. The minute I started straining to cough, they starting pulling on the tube. It wasn't rough coming out, but it seemed so long I wondered if it would ever pop out. When it finally did I coughed for real and then took a deep breath, then looked at Rexanne.

"Hey," I said weakly and hoarsely but with a big smile. She knew I meant, "I love you."

"Hey yourself," she said, smiling back. "Now shut up."

Within a few hours my doctor decided I was breathing on my own just fine, so I was moved out of intensive care.

It was wonderful to be in a normal room with my family and friends all around me. Of course I had plenty of questions about the surgery, including how I ended up with a tube down my throat. Later I realized my breathing troubles during and after surgery probably had something to do with all those troubled nights because of my sleep apnea.

Twelve

NURSE RATCHED IS A MAN

The doting, constant care of the extremely nice nurses in the ICU was a memory. In my regular hospital room, my own personal Nurse Ratched was in charge. Nurse Mildred Ratched, in an Oscar-winning performance by Louise Fletcher in the movie "One Flew Over the Cuckoo's Nest," will go down in screen history as the world's meanest, nastiest nurse. But my Nurse Ratched was not a burly woman who treated me poorly. Instead it was a man who challenged me to start getting better from the first moment he barreled into my room.

He introduced himself and asked me how I was feeling as he zipped from one side of the bed to the other, arranging things exactly the way he wanted them.

"I'm feeling much better now the breathing tube is out and I can finally speak," I whispered, still hoarse.

"Good, now that you can talk, we'll see if you can walk," he replied.

Rexanne and I both gave him a look of terror as he walked out the door.

"Is he serious?" I asked her. "He wants me to start walking already?"

"I don't know," she said, obviously as worried as I was.

"I hope he's not just starting his shift," I told her. "This could be a long twelve hours."

Nurse Ratched returned less than an hour later, and it turned out he was serious about the walking thing. He started moving furniture around in the room, making a clear path from my bed to the door.

"Time to take a little walk," he announced.

"How am I supposed to do that?" I demanded.

"How do you do it at home?" he shot back.

"At home I don't have twenty-nine staples holding a twelve-inch wound together, with an I.V. in my arm and a damn tube in my penis." Nurse Ratched ignored all that, and had me swing my legs over the side of the bed and prop myself up into a sitting position. He grabbed my hands and told me to stand. Once I was up my legs shook a little, but for the most part I was stable. We arranged all the tubes coming from my body so that they wouldn't get caught on anything – especially the catheter. Then he put a second gown on me, reversed so that my huge butt wasn't showing, and I began to walk.

My room was only about twenty feet from the window at the end of the hall. Nurse Ratched told me to walk slowly to the window and back while he changed the bed linens. Surprising myself, I made it to the window and back with ease and wanted to walk a little more.

"Let's go down to the nurses' station," I told Rexanne, who was hovering by my side.

"You sure?" she said.

I nodded, already walking. They were baby steps all the way, but I made it.

"Hello," I said to the nurses, as nonchalantly as I could.

They said hello back and beamed at me. Back in my room, I told Nurse Ratched about my triumph. He was less than impressed. "Next time you can go two laps," he said.

My other excursion that day was a ride in my bed down to the X-ray department to make sure I didn't have any leaks in my stomach. But there was a little problem. My bed was six inches lower than the X-ray table. I had to somehow roll or climb up onto it. I wasn't too concerned. After all, I had already walked to the nurses' station and back. I was wrong. It felt like I was trying to climb a mountain. It seemed like my incision was going to rip apart as I pulled and pushed my self onto the taller table.

After I was settled onto the X-ray table they rewarded me with my first drink of a liquid since the surgery. When they handed me the little cup they told me just to sip a little at a time very slowly. I knew right away that the chalky fluid was no reward; it was more like punishment. After a few minutes of feeling the chalky liquid going through my body like a giant swimming pool slide, it landed in my stomach. When X-rays showed that the liquid didn't leak out of my stomach, they gave me the all-clear and sent me back to my room. The staff also told me that I could start drinking clear liquids. It was definitely easier to slide off the hard X-ray table down onto my soft bed.

When they wheeled me back to my room, I don't know whether I was happier to see the friends waiting for me or Nurse Ratched extending a cup of cool water. It really is amazing how good water can taste after almost 48 hours without a drink. Even though it was only about two ounces, it seemed like a gallon. The nurse gave me a little grin as he walked out the door and said, "I'll be back in a while for a few more laps." I hit the morphine button and talked with my friends until I passed out.

By the time Nurse Ratched returned, I already was on the side of the bed and ready to do my laps. "Great, if you can make it to the side of the bed, you can make it up by yourself," he said. I fell right into his trap.

"How'm I supposed to do that?"

"How would you do it at home?" he replied, like a comedian pouncing on a punch line.

I stared at the floor, determined to get my butt out of that bed. When I finally got myself out of bed, I never even looked in his direction. Rexanne covered my giant butt with another gown and we made our rounds around the nurse's station. Twice!

Thirteen

DAY THREE

After a long day of tests and laps around the nurse's station, I was down for a nice long nap. When I woke up it was about 10 p.m. and my new nurses were on duty. During the shift change Nurse Ratched was replaced by two young female nurses. They were sweet girls and they tended to my every need. I was even lucky enough to have a two-girl sponge bath. When they asked me if I had been given a bath that day, I told them no and they went right to it.

"Here, let us help you out of bed," they cooed.

"No problem, I can do it myself," I said.

"You can?" They seemed incredulous. I told them about my day with Nurse Ratched and how he had gotten me out of bed and doing laps in the hallway, and they were amazed at my progress. I had been thinking Nurse Ratched was solely interested in torturing me, but maybe the guy knew what he was doing by pushing me.

After my nice little sponge bath, it was lights out and I slept well. I woke up the next morning, looked over at Rexanne on her little cot and thought, "She must feel like crap."

It was Sunday morning and she had been by my side since Friday morning. I knew she could not take another night on that cot. She woke up, realized that I had been watching her sleep, and murmured, "Good Morning." It was one of those moments when I really understood how much she loved me and really realized I couldn't live without her.

We watched some Sunday morning TV and then my sponge buddies brought us breakfast – the first dose of Ensure for me and the hospital breakfast for Rexanne. After they served up our hospital delicacy, the gals informed us that their shift was over. When I asked them who was on next, their facial expression explained it all.

Just before lunch, Nurse Ratched was back with more good news: before I could go home, I had to use the bathroom on my own. I didn't even think about the bathroom part of his sentence. I was worried about the going home part.

"Going home?" I asked. "Are you sure you have the right room?" I had been breathing on my own for only about twenty-four hours, and just started to walk. I wasn't ready to be home on my own. No sponge baths. No morphine.

"You're doing fine," he said. "If the doctor says it's OK, you can go home this evening."

In the time it took me to reach for the morphine button, he grabbed the catheter tube and yanked it out like he was starting a lawn mower. All in all, I have to give credit to Nurse Ratched. He was tough but fair, and pushed my buttons only to make me work harder. I had to thank him for that, and eventually I did. But before I left I wanted to get him back. He returned to my room a short while after winning the gold medal in the catheter-jerking competition, and I told him that I thought I could try and use the bathroom. He started clearing a path for me to get to the bathroom as I got myself out of bed. When I reached the bathroom door he was clearly leaving the room, but I gave him a look of confusion. I would need a little help once I got into the bathroom and he was not offering any. I was still four hundred fifty pounds, had twenty-nine staples in my stomach, and I couldn't reach around the mass of fat.

I asked him how I was supposed to do that. Of course he said, "How would you do it at home?"

That would be the last time he spoke those words to me. I walked into the bathroom, used both hands to hold up my hospital gown and let fly. It sure seemed I was aiming for the toilet, but I'm pretty sure I missed a lot, too. When Nurse Ratched returned a few minutes later he looked in the bathroom and turned to me with a disgusted look on his face.

"Well, how are we going to clean this up"? he demanded.

I had been waiting for this.

"Well," I said, "how would you do it at home?"

Before long the doctor came into my room and announced that I was doing amazingly well. He didn't see why I couldn't go home that afternoon.

"No," I protested. "I'm not well enough. Maybe I need one more night here." I didn't think I was ready to give up my morphine button, my tag-team sponge baths and my big comfy hospital bed for a recliner at home.

"You're doing well, and you are ready," the doctor insisted. "You'll be home in a few hours, and you'll be glad to be there."

A few hours later I was in an extra-large wheel chair, holding a pillow across my belly, heading for the exit doors. When the volunteer pushed me through the automatic doors, the air was thickly humid on that late August afternoon. But it was fresh air and it was wonderful. We waited as Rexanne pulled my truck around to pick me up at the curb. Getting in wasn't as difficult as I thought, and we began the twenty-minute drive home.

"Watch the bumps," I begged Rexanne.

When we arrived at the house, my parents and my niece were waiting for us on the front porch, happy to see us. They helped me to my recliner in the living room and had a good dose of liquid Lortab painkiller waiting for me. I slowly drank the shot of medication and tried to hold a conversation until I passed out.

Fourteen

ENSURE...THE BARIATRIC BREAKFAST

I slept on and off during the night and took my medication as needed. I watched TV in between medicated sleep sessions until the rest of the crowd woke up the next morning. You wouldn't believe the number of infomercials on TV at 3 a.m.

While Rexanne was getting ready for work, my Mom asked me if I was ready for breakfast. I told her I was, even though I was not the slightest bit hungry. Really, I wasn't hungry at all. Food never crossed my mind. When she arrived with the two ounces of Ensure I asked her what flavor it was. I had to ask, because on the night of the Fat Saturday party my friends gave me cases and cases of Ensure in every flavor made. My mom had even purchased the cappuccino flavor because she knows how I love coffee in the morning. She told me it was chocolate and I sipped the two ounces for five minutes. It didn't take long to figure out that ice-cold chocolate Ensure was my favorite, and quickly became breakfast, lunch, and dinner.

Over the next couple of days I began a routine of Ensure, liquid Lortab, and walks to and from the bathroom. Eventually, pieces of banana were on my diet. Talk about a taste treat. Then I was allowed a scrambled egg. It didn't settle well at first, but with time was fine. I was officially on the road to soft foods.

By the time my parents left a few days later, I was getting up and down the stairs on my own and walking to the mailbox each morning. I was getting around fairly well, but still sleeping on the recliner. I tried to lie on the bed one evening when Rexanne was home, but stretching those staples was still painful. After more than a week in that recliner I was ready to sleep in my own bed, next to the woman I love. I climbed into bed one night and never slept in that recliner again.

A day or two before it was time to have my staples removed, I noticed a stain on my T-shirt. When I lifted it up I saw that the stain was coming from my incision. I immediately called Rexanne on her cell phone. "I have a leak," I told her.

According to what I had learned, a leak was the worst thing in the world. People die from leaks.

"Call Bobbie Lou," Rexanne told me.

Bobbie Lou is the glue that holds the bariatric program together at East Carolina's Brody School of Medicine. Sure, the doctors are the brilliant folks who save lives, but Bobbie Lou, a nurse and so much more, is the one person we all turn to when we need answers – no matter what the question.

When I called she wasn't available, but she returned my call in less than an hour. She reassured me that it was not a real leak.

"A real leak is internal," she said, "and you just have liquid externally from the incision."

"Why?" I wondered. "Was this a problem?"

"Don't worry, it's fine," she assured me. "Just come in to get the staples removed in a couple of days and we'll check everything out. And don't worry."

Fifteen

PACK! PACK! PACK!

When I arrived at the hospital for my first visit since the surgery, a nurse took my vital signs and weighed me. I had lost twenty pounds in ten days. I was ecstatic. I went to the examination room where Dr. Chapman would check me out. Bobbie Lou took a look at my staples and told me that I had a small hole in my incision – that's what caused the external fluid that had worried me. She told me that my incision was deep, and that sometimes fluid needs to seep out though the incision. She then told me it was better out than in, and she said they were going to remove the staples.

"Uh, Bobbie Lou," I ventured, "maybe we should leave the staples in a little longer to make sure no more little holes pop up."

"It'll be fine," she told me. Another nurse grabbed this staple-remover tool and went to work. I was amazed at how easy and fast the removal of twenty-nine staples went. I thought to myself, "That was pretty simple," Then Dr. Chapman came in and things got a little less simple.

He examined my incision and the small hole inside it. He started pushing on both sides of my stomach with his hands squeezing the two sides together. Ooze came out of the small hole. Without saying a word, he opened a drawer in small medical cabinet behind him and put on the rubber gloves. When he turned back to me holding a long, wooden Q-tip, I knew things were going to get worse.

"Deep incisions like yours often have fluid buildup," he said, "and that fluid has got to get out." Before I knew it, he had turned the Q-tip with the wooden end – not the soft cottony end – facing my stomach. He was going to help drain the fluid. Before I could suggest that we let it drain on its own, he poked another hole in my incision and more ooze came out. I was intrigued and disgusted at the same time as I watched my doctor poke holes into a belly that he had stapled shut ten days earlier. When he figured out that small holes were part of one big one, he played connect the dots and created about a two inch opening. When the ooze started rolling out of my stomach it looked like a scene from the movie "Aliens." I stopped watching, laid my head back and stared at the ceiling.

When it was all said and done, I had three holes in my incision about the size that you could stick a finger in. He told me to expect more to appear over the weekend, and he wanted me back in the office Monday afternoon. Dr. Chapman also told me that I would need to pack the holes with gauze twice a day after I showered and cleaned the wounds. He pulled apart a two-inch by two-inch gauze pad and began pushing it gently into the holes in my incision with the wooden end of the long Q-tip. I never knew how versatile a darn Q-tip could be. Kind of like a shovel, he used it to open up a hole and then to fill it back in again.

When I came out of the exam room Rexanne could tell by the look on my face that I was not a happy camper. I gave her the whole story as we drove toward the coast. She had work in the area, and I decided that a break from house arrest would be good for me. Other than a weekend of packing my wounds and showering twice a day, it wasn't all bad. It was also the first time I was allowed fish in my diet. I remember we went to a local restaurant in Atlantic Beach named Loughry's Landing and I had my first taste of solid food in almost two weeks. The tiny bit of baked fish were delicious, but more importantly, it settled very well in my new stomach.

Monday morning it was time for me to get back to work. My doctors originally wanted me to stay out for three weeks, but that was not going to happen. I had decided long before my surgery that I would go back as soon as I could drive. I said I would just work the morning show, then go home and rest. I remember how tired I was after that first show. I looked forward to getting home, drinking a good shot of Lortab, and sleeping all afternoon. But I still had to go to the doctor for the follow-up.

He confirmed what he had predicted. More holes. In fact, two of the holes had split even more and became one big one. He went right for the gloves and wooden Q-tip, and began excavating my belly again. He looked like he was on a mission as he poked and prodded the thin layer of skin that held the incision together. I quit watching after he showed me how deep the biggest hole was, sticking the eight-inch Q-tip eighty percent of the way into my stomach. I could just see the white cotton part sticking out.

After several minutes of exclaiming how much fluid he was draining from the wounds, he announced, "That should do it." When I finally glanced down again, my incision looked like Swiss cheese and I began to roll my eyes and groan. This time, when he turned back from the medical cabinet he brought a lot more gauze and told me that things were going to be harder now.

"You'll need to change the packing in the wounds three times a day," he said.

My routine became cleaning and packing the wounds in the morning after I showered, in the afternoon following work, and finally just before bed. Dr. Chapman suggested a home health nurse come to my house to pack and unpack the holes.

"No, I'll do it myself," I said.

"Are you sure?" he pressed. "The holes are going to take several weeks to heal."

I nodded and watched him carefully as he began to pack the holes to make sure I did it the same way. The two-inch gauze pads had grown to the bigger four-inch size and the largest hole took several of them. When I left the office that day I had several hospital bags full of gauze, tape, and Q-tips. The office staff told me the supply should last a couple of days until I could get to the drug store. I knew it was going to be several long, long weeks.

Sixteen

BABY PUKE

I did everything exactly as the doctor instructed and the holes healed in about six weeks. By then I had lost fifty pounds and was eating all solid foods. My weekly exams were going very well. I was even getting into an exercise routine at the gym three days a week. However, I still had a few diet lessons to learn.

One evening we were with friends at one of our favorite spots, a Friday night tradition at the beach, named The Beach Tavern. I decided to try one of their famous chicken wings. After all, I had been eating chicken and beef for several weeks and didn't have any problem with it. Even though they were fairly small, I still knew I would only be able to eat a couple.

The wings were fried, but not breaded, and after a couple of small bites, the first seemed to go down OK. Even though I was eating slowly, by the time I had taken two bites of the second wing, it felt like I was full up to my throat. Then the pain started in my stomach and I thought if I just stopped for a few minutes it would pass like the times before. Everyone knew something was wrong and Rexanne commented that I didn't look so good. I got up to walk around a bit, but felt worse. I walked quickly past the table and told Rexanne I had to leave but would be right back. Outside, I started to walk in the direction of our trailer, only a couple of blocks away. I knew what was about to happen, and I wasn't looking forward to it. After only a few steps, I felt the food coming up and quickly moved toward a trashcan. I leaned over and started to gag, then heaved a little as my eyes teared up. When the chicken wing and half started to come up it felt like an entire turkey, but what came up turned out to be a surprisingly small amount of re-gurgitation. You couldn't put it in the palm of a child's hand. (Not that you would.) Once I realized no body parts came up with the chicken and I was still intact, I started to get mad. All the drama for that tiny amount of throwup? It looked liked an infant had spit up.

From what the hospital had told me, I was under the impression that if I ate too much my whole insides might come up. They had been using scare tactics and they had worked. Later when Dr. Chapman and I talked and laughed about the incident, he told me the skin from that dreaded chicken wing could not pass through the tiny opening between my new pouch and small intestine. No matter, because that incident left a lasting impression on me. Today, almost three years later, I still won't eat fried chicken.

During the next few months I learned more about my new stomach and had my first experience with dumping. When we were on a trip to Savannah, Ga. with our friends I decided to have a beer while play-ing golf with my buddy David Godwin. I had sipped on a beer a few times before, but nothing like the way I could guzzle them down before surgery. After the first beer went down OK I tried another and I was feeling a little tipsy. A few hours later in downtown Savannah, hanging out at a local brewpub, we decided to try their five-beer sampler. The samples weren't full beers, just five small glasses of the bar's own home brew, about three ounces each. I sipped on them for a while but never finished them. I knew then that beer wasn't for me anymore. Besides, I had already found a new substitute for the beer. Wine had no carbon-ation and was something I had always enjoyed, but it had never been my alcohol of choice. Beer was.

But that night in Savannah I learned the hard way that my new body, more than sixty pounds lighter, couldn't handle alcohol the way it used to. I don't really remember going back to the hotel at the end of a late night of what I thought were a few drinks. What I do remember was waking up at about five –o'clock in the morning feeling wet. I couldn't understand what was wrong. I just knew that I had to use the bathroom. When I turned the bathroom light on, my boxer shorts were soaked, but I still hadn't a clue what was going on. As I walked back to the bed I started putting things together. You guessed it. I had wet the bed like a four-year-old. I made the mistake of telling my friends about it when I explained why I was laying off the beer, and you don't want to know how much crap I took from them.

There were other forms of dumping and body changes that I had to figure out on my own. One morning about six months after surgery, Rexanne and I were at breakfast and I decided try some pancakes. Even though I didn't eat much, it was all that I had. The small amount of pancakes filled me up quickly and I didn't even consider the fact that I hadn't eaten any protein. A few hours later I was in the shower when I started feeling incredibly dizzy and my heart began to race. When I got out and dried off I told Rexanne that I didn't feel good at all and held out my hand so she could see it shaking.

I went to lie down, and after about thirty minutes I felt fine.

This happened a few more times over the next month, so I told my doctor about it. They did blood work to look for anything suspect, but the tests all came back fine. Katrina, my dietitian and the co-author of this book, helped me figure it out. She told me to write down the foods that I had just eaten the next time I had an episode. I quickly learned that my dumping occurred after eating meals that were high in carbohydrates and had little to no protein.

It's amazing how your body can teach you behavior modification. I now know I can't eat pancakes alone. I should eat protein first at every meal in combination with some carbohydrates. I can have sweets, like cake or ice cream occasionally, but only a few bites and after I have eaten a good source of protein. When I follow those guidelines it's easy and life is good.

Seventeen

CLOTHES HORSE

By November, a little over four months since the surgery, I had lost one hundred pounds. I already looked like a totally different person and the weight was still falling off every week. By the time my first-year checkup came around, I had lost one hundred and sixty pounds and was right on track with the weight loss. The doctors estimate you will lose eighty percent of your estimated weight loss within the first twelve months and the remaining twenty percent the next year.

Everything was so much easier than before. I could work out on a regular basis with little effort. My back stopped hurting and I slept through the night without the use of a breathing machine. I crossed my legs everywhere I went and yes, I even sat in booths at restaurants. When the morning show took listeners to a theme park that summer, I rode every roller coaster in the park twice. That is when I became an addict; not to drugs, but clothes. Rexanne had officially given me the title "clothes whore."

I went from a size sixty in the waist to a forty-two and was wearing a double-X shirt. I could shop anywhere I wanted to and I did, often. As my weight continued to drop, I continued to shop. Not in big and tall stores, but at Gap, Hilfiger, Abercrombie, and more. If it had a name brand other than "Huge," I bought it. My addiction to T-shirts was the worst. I am now the proud owner of more than one hundred T-shirts. For the first time I'm wearing T-shirts from every regular hangout and every country we've visited because, let me tell you, not a lot of places carried a XXXXXL. Of course, as I lost weight I needed new clothes and smaller sizes, so we had a really big tax write-off from the clothes I donated to charity.

During our monthly support group meetings, I found out that I was not the only person wearing the "clothes whore" title. We all had the same stories of weight loss and new wardrobes. It seemed like everyone could remember the exact dates and clothing purchases they made for every size dropped. The monthly support group meetings are a great time to learn facts and share stories. It was also where I met my future co-author, dietitian and friend, Katrina Segrave.

The day I met Katrina or "Kat," as just about everyone calls her, I was chatting with some other post-op patients as we waited for our monthly support group to begin. For the most part, it's not too hard to spot who's there for the meeting, but sometimes people surprise you. From the minute Kat walked in, I was pretty sure this tall blonde was not a post-op patient. I was right. Kat was there to talk to our group about the benefits of yoga and exercise. She was carrying some apparatus in one hand and some papers in the other. I complimented her on her shoes. (Living with Rexanne, I have come to appreciate a woman who knows good shoes, and to know that they appreciate a man who notices.)
I nodded to the thing in her hand. "I don't know what you're planning to do with that contraption, but sign me up!"
She laughed, thanked me for the shoe recognition, and informed me that she was a registered dietitian, exercise specialist, and yoga instructor … and that "contraption" was an aid for learning to stand on my head, if I was still interested. Stand on my head? Hey, not long ago I couldn't cross my legs. Sign me up.

The next week I scheduled my first nutrition consultation. I learned so much during that meeting. I knew right then that Kat and I made a great team. We teamed up to fine-tune my diet and even began some personal training. Kat made it her mission not only to give me a great workout each time, but to teach me how to kick my own butt as my fitness level improved. She's so into health and physical fitness, words can't describe it. She's like Dr. Frankenstein creating a new specimen; the more work she puts into it, the crazier things get. And the better things get. There were some days I'd wake up feeling parts of my body I didn't even know existed. I wasn't complaining, though. I was learning so much and the results were irrefutable.

Eighteen

NIP! TUCK!

About a year after surgery, I started to notice a little bulge in the middle of my stomach. I would like to think that it was the making of a tightly ripped stomach from thousands of the crunches Kat had me doing. No such luck. What I dreamt was muscle and the beginning of a six-pack turned out to be a hernia. You can imagine how I felt, after all of the stomach related problems I had been through, when I was told that I needed surgery again. Dr. Chapman said he would have to place a mesh patch under my skin to fix the hernia and make sure it would not re-emerge.

I had been thinking about a tummy tuck for several months, but never really pursued it. I even met with one of the hospital's plastic surgeons for an initial consultation. He explained to me the ins and outs of surgery and told me how much it would cost.

I had been saving for a tummy tuck since my first surgery, so the shock didn't knock me off the exam table. But now I had a good reason to step things up a bit. I knew that the original plastic surgeon I met with would be with the practice only for a few more months, so I had to go back and meet my new choice for a plastic surgeon, Dr. Zeri. He urged me to wait until I lost more weight. But I was determined to have both surgeries, hernia and plastic, at the same time. I would later regret that demand. Dr. Zeri made it clear to me that while the tummy tuck would look good, there would still be some fat around the love handles. What did I care? Up until that point I had love steering wheels, not handles.

This surgery was also scheduled on a Friday morning, and things went exactly the same as before. We were in the waiting room just a few minutes, then into the prep area for another belly shave. Rexanne came back in for a quick visit before the staff took me into the holding area. But this time, the holding area was more like art class. Dr. Zeri spent the better part of a half-hour drawing on me with a marker. By the time he was done, my stomach and sides looked like a roadmap. I studied them as the nurse came in to inject something into my IV line. A few minutes later I was rolling down the hallway, although I don't ever remember making it to the operating room.

The first time I regained consciousness, Dr. Zeri was waking me to inform me that the surgery went so well that they decided to do liposuction to my sides; the love handles were gone. I was still really out of it and I could not understand why he was waking me up in the operating room to tell me this. However, the last thing he told me was clear as a bell.

"You're going to experience a little more discomfort than originally planned," he warned.

"A little discomfort" is a doctor's way of saying that it was going to hurt like hell. The second time I came out of dreamland I was in the recovery room. The doctor was there, and so was a little discomfort. I felt like I had taken the worst beating in my life.

After a little while in recovery, they wheeled me into my room. Rexanne was waiting for me. Of course, it only took a few moments before Rexanne was ready for a look. She told me that Dr. Zeri had filled her in on the liposuction and the added discomfort. But he didn't tell her how nasty it was going to look. I had already checked it out myself, so I warned her in advance about how bad things looked before I lowered the sheet. At first I just showed her the incision on my stomach where they fixed the hernia. It looked great. Then I slowly moved the sheet to one side so she could get a good look at the liposuction. The look on her face said it all. It looked like I had been beaten with a tire iron on both my sides and parts of my lower back.

The pain I experienced over the next few days in the hospital can only be described as pure hell. There is no way to sugarcoat it or try to convince you otherwise – it hurt non-stop. When I had to climb back in bed after the first time getting up, I'm sure they heard me on the other side of the hospital. Morphine became a very good friend of mine. There was a constant pulling on the incision that went from the middle of my chest, all around my belly button, and then around both side of my waistline.

When I asked the doctor how many stitches I had, he just said "Hundreds." For three weeks after surgery I had several tubes coming out of my lower incision to drain fluid from the healing wound. The tubes had to be emptied and the amount had to be measured daily to be sure the proper amount of fluid drained. I remember cutting holes in the pockets of my pants so I could bring the tubes through the holes and let them rest in my pockets while I was at work. If the tubes got hung on something and pulled on the few stitches holding them in, everyone within earshot would know it.

With every passing week the doctor would remove a couple tubes as they stopped draining. Once the final drainage tube was removed, I was given the all-clear. Everything has been great ever since. For the first six months I would get an occasional pulling or tightness from the scars, but it was a small price to pay to be rid of the flab hanging in my lap. Before the plastic surgery I was in a size forty-two pants; afterward I immediately dropped four inches around my waist and now wear a size thirty-eight and a thirty-six in some pants.

When people ask me if I'd do it again, I tell them absolutely. In fact my next goal is to have plastic surgery to have my "man boobs" removed. That should be fun.

Nineteen

THE NEW YOU – AND ME

Three years post-op, I am definitely a different person. I'd like to think I'm smaller and a little wiser. My weight has not changed by more than five pounds in the past year and I recently ran in my second 5-K road race, cutting my time down by seven minutes. Who knows, maybe I can participate in a triathlon one day. One thing I know for certain, I enjoy my new weight. I will never get tired of hearing people say how good I look or seeing the amazement on someone's face when I show them my picture before surgery, which I keep in my wallet to this day.

Now that I know what it's like to be thin, I don't ever want that to change. However, I know it's possible to gain weight. I've heard stories from other patients who've gained some or all of their weight back, and it really scares me. I know that keeping my weight off means a lot more than simply eating smaller portions; I must make appropriate food choices at every meal. The new stomach pouch that our wonderful surgeons have created for us is just "a tool." Tools only work when we know how to use them properly.

So I've teamed up with the most knowledgeable person I know, my co-author, Katrina Segrave. She's an expert on nutrition and fitness and she's passionate about showing you how to reach your goal weight and – more importantly – how to maintain it. In the chapters to come, Katrina will give you an "owner's manual" for weight loss success.

If you're like me, sometimes you need to be slapped right in the face with what needs to be done. That's exactly what Katrina is going to do. She'll explain to you, in laymen's terms, basic nutrition and how to make the right food choices. She has included a four-week sample meal plan, recipe ideas and a variety of exercise programs you can use in the gym or at home. We will even demonstrate how to properly perform some of the core exercises discussed with pictures of me in action at the gym.

So if you never received nutrition support from your surgeon, your eating habits are slipping, or you aren't getting the results you'd like from your current exercise program, the next section of this book is for you. We will empower you with the knowledge and skills to maintain the weight loss you've waited your entire life to achieve.

I've done it with Kat's help, and so can you.

PATIENT SUCCESS STORIES

Jerry and Rexanne

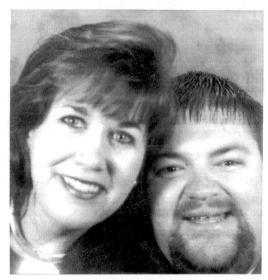

**Photo booth in the mall while
Chistmas shopping in 1994.**

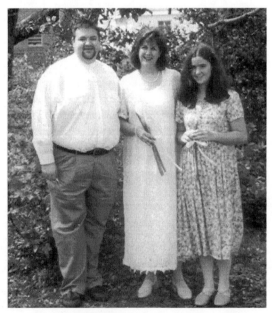

**March 29th 1996, our wedding day,
a little ove 350 lbs.**

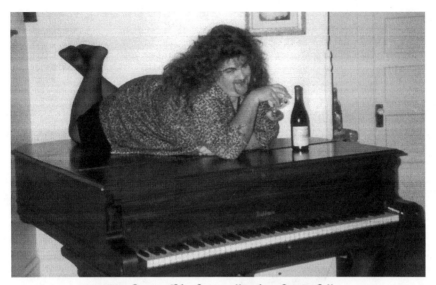

**Goofing off before a "Relay for Life"
Woman-less beauty pageant. I won!**

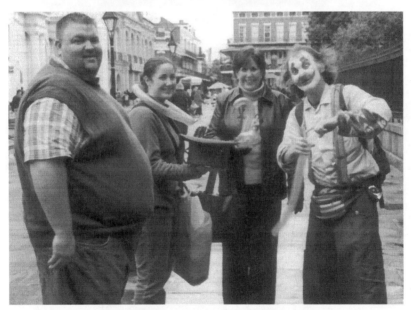

Living LARGE in New Orleans!

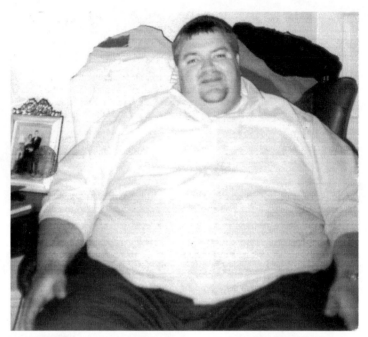

2002 – One week before surgery – 450 pounds.

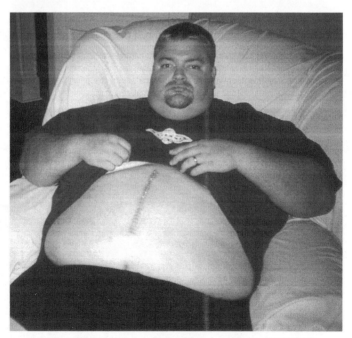

Three days post-op and 29 staples – WOW!

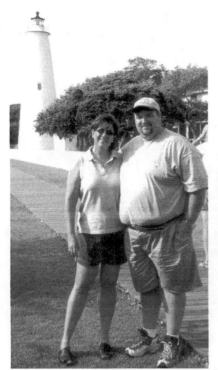
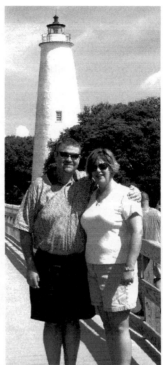

Light House on Okracoke Island, NC
Pre-op then post op.

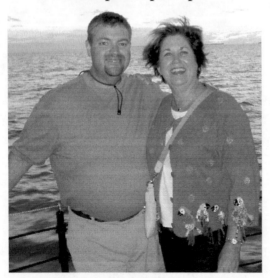

Vacation in Key West... 245 lbs

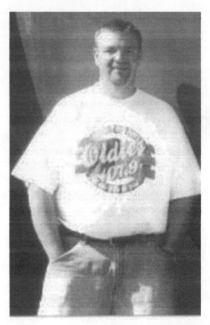

2004 – Just being a radio guy…down 210 pounds.

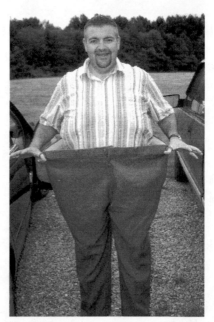

**2005 – Standing in my former size 60 pants…
now almost half my pre-op weight.**

Meet my brother Craig...
pre-op weight 353 lbs.

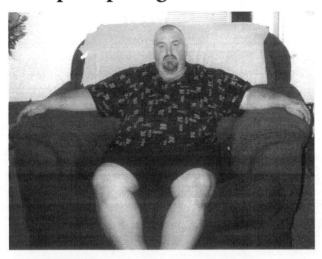

The man who could woof down two bologna sandwiches in 6.8 seconds, now weighs in at 205 lbs. I am more proud of him for making this decision than he will ever know.

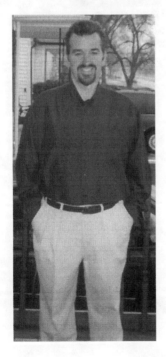

Martha Carter

Surgery Date: May 2003
Pre-Op Weight: 342 pounds
Current Weight: 145 lbs pounds

Martha's Motivation to Maintain

Health! Martha's medical issues were jeopardizing her physical and emotional well being. Since surgery she has been able to tackle any health issues head on and now enjoys activities in her life that she never thought possible again.

Having gone from a size 24/26 to a size 8/10, Martha uses new clothes as another motivator to keep the weight off.

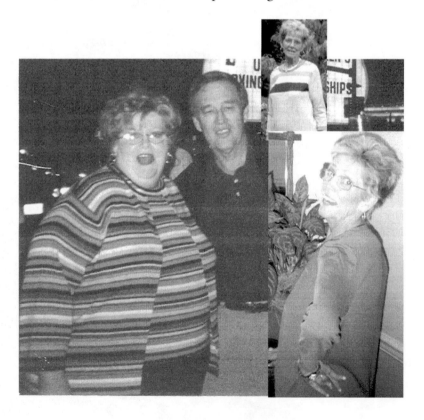

Wendy Cunningham

Surgery Date: June 2001
Pre-Op Weight: 450 pounds
Pounds Lost: 200

Life Before Surgery:

"I would wake up in agony because of the pain in my knees. A walker was kept beside my bed to assist my first steps of the day. It took every ounce of energy I had just to get up, shower and dress. Then I had to work 8 hours. My life had come to a screeching halt. My joints were on the way out and I was literally looking at life in a wheel chair.

"I went from being a 'side show' to a 'socially acceptable plus size.' My self-esteem is back and I live my life to the fullest! I have lost 200 pounds and have a new lease on life. I don't believe I will ever be a thin person but that's okay; I can walk again!

"People are amazed at simple gestures that I will never again take for granted. You have no idea what my life was like, if you could have only walked one day in my shoes.

"To be honest you probably couldn't do it!"

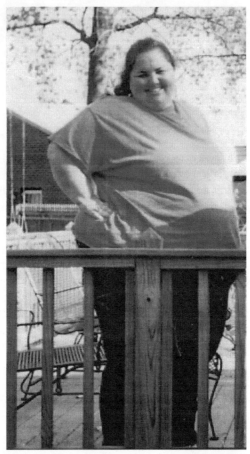

1994 – "About 375 pounds, here; not my heaviest weight."

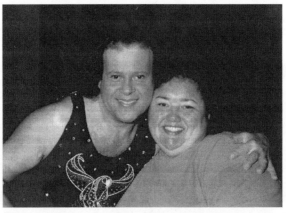

1999 – On the "Cruise to Lose" with Richard Simmons - 400 pounds

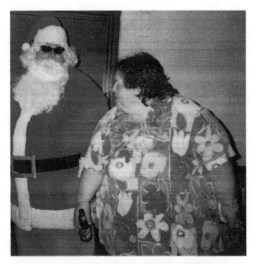

December 2000 – 425 pounds – "I should have been Santa!"

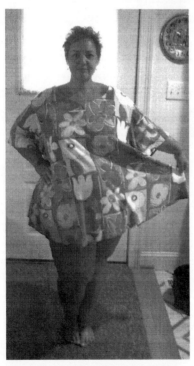

June 2005 – 250 pounds - "Feeling sassy in a dress that is too big, now! The hips and thighs will be history after plastic surgery scheduled for later this year."

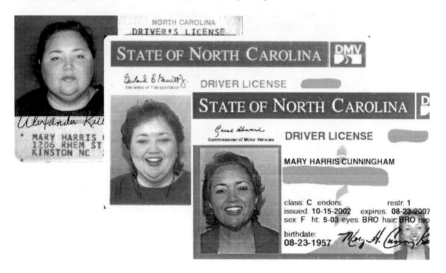

"My weight documented by the state of North Carolina. The first two driver's license pictures were in 1993 and in 1997 at an approximate weight of 400 pounds. The last license picture was taken in 2002, about 14 months after my surgery and 200 pounds lighter. This was the first picture I had seen of myself since losing weight. Standing in the D.M.V. office that day, I honestly did not recognize myself. I immediately handed the card back to the clerk stating that he had given me someone else's license!"

Billy Dunn

Surgery Date: October 19th, 2004
Pre-Op Weight: 340
Current Weight: 200

Billy's Motivation for Choosing Surgery:

Both of my parents passed away at an early age because of heart problems brought on by obesity. I enjoy my kids; I want to do everything I can to stay healthy so I'll be around to spoil my grandchildren… like grandparents are supposed to!

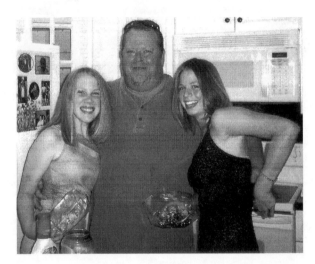

**2004 – 340 pounds – Billy with his daughter Kelly
(on right) and a friend.**

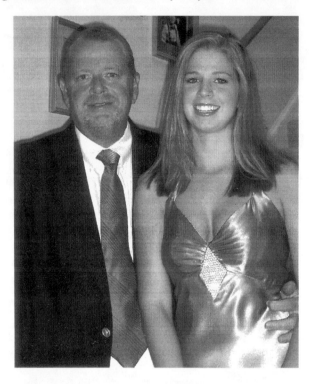

**2005 – All smiles and 113 pounds lighter
– Billy with his daughter, Kelly.**

Lu Ann Sullivan

Pre-Op Weight: 291 pounds
Current Weight: 140 pounds

Lu Ann is a beautiful person, inside and out! You can count on seeing her at ECU's monthly patient support group meeting, which is where Jerry and Katrina both came to know her as "friend." Lu Ann epitomizes the "success-story" patient and goes the extra mile to inspire and encourage others considering gastric bypass surgery.

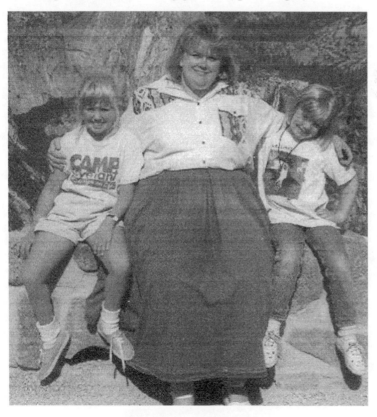

Lu Ann with her two daughters.

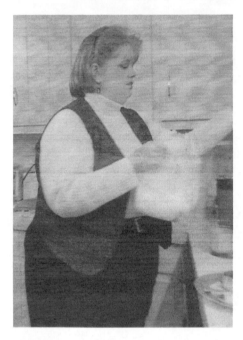

The night before her surgery, at just shy of 300 pounds.

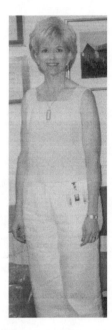

Lu Ann, at 135 pounds... Actually tring to *gain* weight back to 140 pounds where she feels the healthiest.

Dena Horne

Surgery Date: August 19, 2004
Pre-Op Weight: 315 pounds
Current Weight: 159 pounds

Dena says her biggest motivation for keeping the weight off is her hope for having children. Before surgery she was unable to conceive, but today doctors say it's possible. Good luck, Dena! We just know you're going to be a fabulous mother!

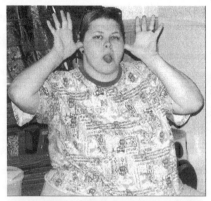

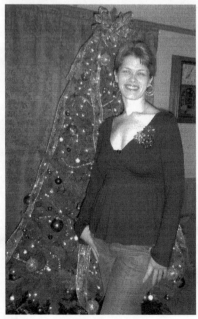

Debbie Bailey

Surgery Date: August 6, 2004
PreOp Weight: 460 pounds
Current weight: 233 pounds

Debbie says "Thank You" for a wonderful new life!

"Without the surgery, I think I would have died in 2 or 3 years! I had sleep apnea, high blood pressure, acid reflux, high cholesterol, cellulitis, chronic lupus flare-ups and many other health problems. I was taking 10 different medications daily, including prednisone which caused even more weight gain. Honestly, I couldn't even walk more than a few steps without becoming severely short of breath. Life was a tremendous struggle.

"Today, I'm happy to go to the YMCA where I now walk on the treadmill for 40 minutes – non-stop! I also use a variety of other cardio machines and am even working weight training into the mix. I'm down from 10 pills to just 2 per day and my health has improved tremendously. Life has so much to offer… it's truly wonderful. Thank you, Dr. Chapman!"

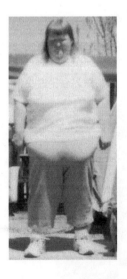
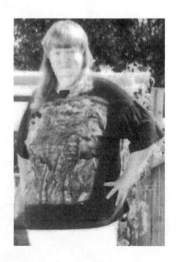

Donna Carter

Gastric Bypass Program Coordinator
Village Surgical Associates
Fayetteville, North Carolina

Surgery Date: June 19, 2002
Pre-op Weight: 300 pounds
Current Weight: 148 pounds

Words of Wisdom from Donna

"Two and a half years after surgery my weight loss began to plateau. Six months later I had not lost another pound and I began to wonder whether or not I would reach my goal weight. After my nutrition consultation with Katrina, I actually increased my calories! By eating three regular meals, using "the plate method," I lost seven more pounds over the next few months …. it was great! The best part is I have kept the weight off and have never felt better. This experience taught me that surgery is only part of the equation. Today, I tell patients about the importance of nutrition for reaching a maintaining a healthy weight after surgery."

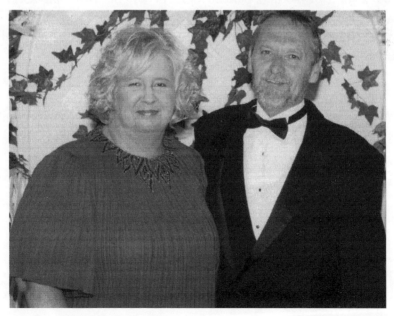

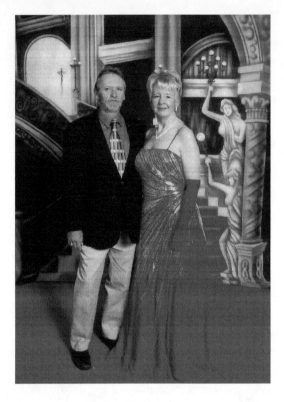

Today, some of Donna's patients don't believe her when she tells them she is a post-gastric-bypass-patient. She keeps before and after pictures in her office to share with doubting patients… and she smiles inside as she shares her amazing story.

Foreword

I met with Registered Dietitian and Exercise Specialist Katrina Segrave in 2002 to discuss adding nutrition and exercise support for our pre-and-post-operative bariatric patients. Katrina tells me today that it was a statement I made during that first meeting that inspired her to author this book. I had stated, "I hope you can help us determine why we are seeing many patients re-gain varying amounts of weight by two to three years post-op." Truly she has answered that question for all of us within the pages of this book.

Katrina completes a critical piece of the weight loss equation for people who have had or are planning to have gastric bypass surgery. For the first time she presents specific diet strategies to ensure successful weight loss and the maintenance of a healthy body weight. With easy to read chapters, she takes the mystery out of following an appropriate post-op diet and dispels the myths about "good foods" vs. "bad foods," portion sizes, dumping, grazing, liquid calories and much, much more.

In addition, there are ideas for getting physically active, staying compliant and maximizing your results from exercise. With four weeks of sample meals and a series of sample cardiovascular and resistance training programs, Katrina takes the guess work out of ensuring your post-operative success. This book is a "must read' for all post-op patients and anyone considering weight loss surgery.

Dr. Kenneth G. MacDonald, Jr., MD, FACS
Chief of Gastrointestinal Surgery,
Director of Surgical Obesity Program,
and Professor of Surgery
East Carolina Univesity
The Brody School of Medicine

Twenty

NUTRITION 101

Introduction

It's normal to have a lot of questions about what to eat following weight loss surgery. I'm often asked, "How many calories will I be eating? How many grams of fat can I have? How much protein do I need? Is it true that I can never eat sugar again? What about net carbs?" It's enough to make your head spin!

A standardized diet for people who've had gastric bypass surgery does not currently exist. Nutrition is a dynamic field; dietitians are continually researching and discovering new things. During my first year of consulting with bariatric patients, I found myself giving pretty general nutrition advice, avoiding specific recommendations for protein, carbohydrate, fat and calories because more specific information was not available. But over time I began to see a pattern in the diets of patients with the most successful weight loss and those who were able to maintain the weight they lost.

My goal in writing this part of the book is to give you the benefit of what I have learned and what I am continuing to learn through working with my patients. I want to empower you with the tools to reach and maintain your goal weight. The guidelines I will be sharing with you in the following chapters are based on subjective data from a sample of more than 2,000 patients seen through my practice in combination with the most current research available.

In the chapters to come, I'll identify food sources of protein, carbohydrate and fat and specific guidelines for each of these nutrients. I will also discuss nutritional supplements and special considerations such as: dumping, nausea, diarrhea, hair loss, depression, weight loss plateaus, drinking alcohol, caffeine and eating out. I have done my best to keep the information simple, yet explain the reasoning behind the guidelines given.

If you prefer a simple bottom line approach, you might want to fast forward to Chapters 24 and 25: "Your Owner's Manual – Six Guidelines for Success" and "Keeping it Simple: Your Eating Plan is as Easy as 1, 2, 3." These chapters summarize the key behavior changes essential to your long-term success, and they will help you progress quickly with information that is simple and easy to apply.

The anecdotes in this book are based on true stories and positive outcomes from my patients and are ones you'll undoubtedly relate to. While there are many different styles of learning -- each reader will have his own objectives for this book -- please look through the exercises in each chapter. You'll find useful tools throughout the book, such as tips for decreasing food cravings, advice on overcoming emotional eating, and strategies for minimizing the dumping syndrome and maximizing weight loss. Although there are dozens of exercises, choose only one or two to start you on your way. As you make your way in those areas, select a couple more.

I've included a chapter on exercise. You will find a variety of sample programs to help you increase your physical activity and continue progressing as your fitness level improves. There are also many ideas for enhancing your level of motivation and keeping exercise fun.

Always follow the guidelines your surgeon, dietitian and medical care team have given you. Use the information provided in this book as a reference while experimenting with what works best for you.

Diet and exercise habits are like any other habit. Just when you feel you have finally mastered a behavior change, you may find yourself backsliding. Be patient with yourself and take it one day at a time. As you commit to practicing the guidelines in this book on a regular basis, and make note of the positive results that you experience, you will embrace effective weight management. You will truly make peace with your body for life.

In This Chapter
- Identify food sources of carbohydrate, protein and fat.
- Understand the guidelines for balancing these three nutrients at each meal.
- Recognize heart healthy sources of dietary fat and which fats to avoid.

Key Words to Know
- *dumping syndrome:* the rapid emptying of food contents from your stomach into the small intestine.
- *empty calories:* foods that have a lot of calories, but little nutritional value (e.g. a donut.)
- *nutrients-dense foods:* foods that are relatively low in calories and rich in nutrients such as fiber, vitamins, minerals and antioxidants (e.g. fruit and vegetables.)

The Basics

Creating appropriate meals after surgery requires a good understanding of the three building blocks: carbohydrate, protein and fat. These are the nutrients your body uses for fuel. The balance of nutrients in your diet has a powerful impact on how long you feel satisfied after eating, whether or not you experience the dumping syndrome, and your ability to lose weight and keep it off. The recommendations in this book are based on an approximate calorie distribution of:
- 32 percent carbohydrate
- 35 percent protein
- 33 percent fat

By eating a balance of protein, carbohydrate and fat in each meal you will minimize your chances of dumping, prevent early return of hunger and keep your overall calorie intake down. You are more likely to get the necessary nutrition you need because no foods are over emphasized or completely eliminated. And because many of your favorite foods can be included within this framework you are less likely to feel deprived. The old adage, "everything in moderation" truly does apply here.

Almost all of the foods we eat contain a mixture of protein, carbohydrate and fat. For the purposes of this program, I'll categorize foods according to the most significant nutrient they contain. The original food guide pyramid, created in 1992 by the U. S. Department of Agriculture and the U. S. Department of Health & Human Services, is a good visual tool to use when learning to look at your foods in this new way (See Table 20.1.)

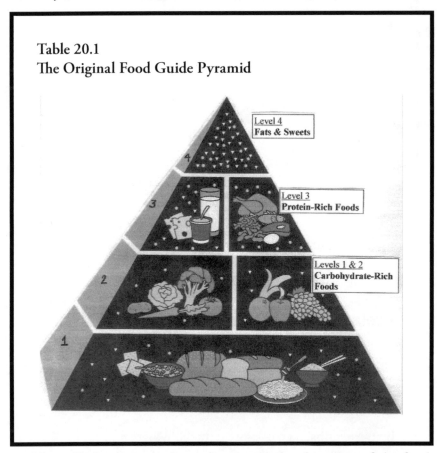

Table 20.1
The Original Food Guide Pyramid

Level 4
Fats & Sweets

Level 3
Protein-Rich Foods

Levels 1 & 2
Carbohydrate-Rich Foods

Note: To learn more about the new, updated version of the food guide pyramid, see Appendix D and visit www.mypyramid.com. To learn more about the bariatric food guide pyramid, see Appendix L.

Carbohydrates

The bottom two levels of the food guide pyramid represent foods that are rich in carbohydrate. These include all starchy foods like bread, muffins, bagels, rice, cereal, pasta and crackers (Level 1), as well as all fruit and vegetables (Level 2). Non-starchy vegetables like green beans, broccoli and salad greens (see Appendix B) have significantly less carbohydrate than fruit and starchy vegetables like potatoes, corn and peas (see Appendix C.) However, all fruit and vegetables are a source of carbohydrate. You will learn appropriate portion sizes for starchy and non-starchy carbohydrates to maximize your weight loss.

Protein

Protein-rich foods are represented on the third level of the food guide pyramid and include: all meats (e.g. fish, chicken, pork, ground beef, steak, roast beef, deli meat and breakfast meats), eggs, egg substitutes, nuts, nut butters (e.g. peanut butter, almond butter, etc.), tofu, cheese, cottage cheese, yogurt, soy-based cheese and meat substitutes. Protein may make up a larger portion of the meals on this plan than you're used to. We'll talk more about this in Chapter 23.

When choosing meat substitutes or dairy-free choices, be sure to read the food label for protein and total carbohydrate content. Some products like veggie burgers or rice milk may not have a significant source of protein and may be a hidden source of carbohydrates.

The Tip of the Pyramid: Fats and Sweets

At the top of the pyramid (Level 4) you will find a collective array of many people's favorite food groups: fat and sugar. Sweets fall into a category often referred to as "other carbohydrates" or "empty calories." These foods are concentrated sources of carbohydrate and calories, yet they lack many of the important vitamins and minerals found in the carbohydrates at the base of the food guide pyramid.

These foods should be avoided during your initial weight loss phase because your food intake is most limited at this time. Filling up on sweets and other empty calories would crowd out more nutrient dense foods at a time when you are already very nutritionally challenged. As you reach your goal weight, some foods from this category may be included in your maintenance diet; however, choose them sparingly and be sure to subtract the grams of carbohydrate from your total carbohydrate budget for that meal. We will discuss specific budgets for protein, carbohydrate and fat in Chapter 24.

Fat

You may be surprised at the amount of fat included in this program because in the past you've probably experimented with very low fat diets. Keep in mind that dietary fat does ***not*** equal body fat. Dietary fat plays an important role in weight loss. Along with protein, the fat we eat helps us feel more satisfied after a meal. You don't have to count every little gram of fat you put in your mouth. When you learn the general guidelines for balancing protein and carbohydrate, you will find it easier to moderate your fat intake without much effort.

Choosing Heart Healthy Fats

Some dietary fat is essential for basic body functions such as transporting the fat soluble vitamins A, D, E and K, making hormones and cell membranes, providing energy and maintaining healthy skin. However, when it comes to heart health, not all fats are created equal. There are three basic types of fat in food: monounsaturated, polyunsaturated and saturated fats. The healthiest fats are monounsaturated and polyunsaturated. Monounsaturated fats help lower harmful LDL and total cholesterol levels and are highest in almonds, avocadoes and oils such as olive, canola and peanut. Polyunsaturated fats help lower total cholesterol and are found in nuts, nut butters, seeds and plant oils such as safflower, sunflower, corn and soybean. Other "good for you fats" include omega-3 fatty acids present in flaxseed, tofu and walnuts, as well as cold-water fish like salmon, tuna, sardines and mackerel.

Saturated fats are those that are solid at room temperature. Lard, for instance, is a saturated fat, where, olive oil is unsaturated. Saturated fats raise your levels of unhealthy LDL cholesterol and increase the risk for heart disease and stroke. These fats are found primarily in animal products such as whole milk, butter, meat and palm & coconut oils. The current dietary reference intakes report doesn't set specific levels for saturated fat, however the recommendation is to eat as little as possible.

"Trans-fatty acids" is a term you may have heard but aren't sure what they are. These are fats that do not occur naturally but are created by adding hydrogen to liquid oil. Food manufacturers often use hydrogenated oils in processed foods like crackers, chips and cookies to increase the food's shelf life. The problem is that solid hydrogenated fat acts like saturated fat in the body, raising bad LDL cholesterol and increasing your risk for heart disease. Effective January 1, 2006 the FDA required all food manufacturers to include trans-fats on the nutrition facts label, making it easier for consumers to identify heart healthy products. Read ingredient labels and avoid products that list "hydrogenated" or "partially hydrogenated" oils as one of the first ingredients.

Comparison of Dietary Fats

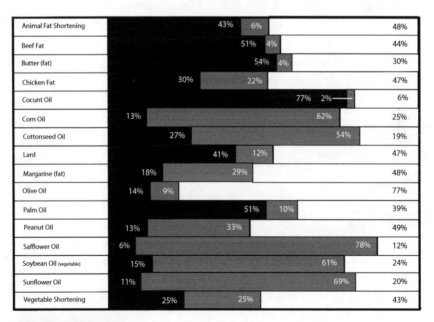

	Saturated Fats	Polyunsaturated Fats	Monounsaturated Fats
Animal Fat Shortening	43%	6%	48%
Beef Fat	51%	4%	44%
Butter (fat)	54%	4%	30%
Chicken Fat	30%	22%	47%
Cocunt Oil	77%	2%	6%
Corn Oil	13%	62%	25%
Cottonseed Oil	27%	54%	19%
Lard	41%	12%	47%
Margarine (fat)	18%	29%	48%
Olive Oil	14%	9%	77%
Palm Oil	51%	10%	39%
Peanut Oil	13%	33%	49%
Safflower Oil	6%	78%	12%
Soybean Oil (vegetable)	15%	61%	24%
Sunflower Oil	11%	69%	20%
Vegetable Shortening	25%	25%	43%

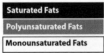

Saturated Fats
Polyunsaturated Fats
Monounsaturated Fats

Bottom Line: One gram of fat has 9 calories, a little more than twice the calories of protein or carbohydrate. Thus moderating your fat intake at each meal is essential in helping you achieve successful weight loss and reduce the risk of stomach discomfort associated with a high fat meal. A good guideline is to limit your fat intake to **10-15 grams per meal** and choose mostly monounsaturated and polyunsaturated fat sources.

Post-Chapter Exercises:

- *Exercise One:* List what you ate for breakfast every morning this week. Next to each item, write whether it was a carbohydrate, fat or protein-rich food.
- *Exercise Two:* Practice reading food labels (see Appendix M, "Anatomy of a food label") and using the dietary exchanges (see Appendix A, B and C) to tally your grams of carbohydrate, fat and protein at each meal.
- *Exercise Three:* Choose heart healthy fats like nuts & seeds, peanut butter, almond butter, avocadoes and olive & canola oil. When reading food labels look for grams of total fat and saturated fat; choose products that contain the smallest percentage of fat from trans and saturated sources.

Twenty-one

A CARB IS A CARB IS A CARB ...

In This Chapter
- Understand the importance of counting total carbohydrate grams, not just grams of sugar, for preventing the dumping syndrome and maximizing weight loss.
- Understand glycemic index, net carbs and sugar alcohols.
- Identify and compare various artificial sweeteners
- Consider the role of fiber and identify fiber-rich foods.

Key Words to Know
- *glycemic index, or GI:* A ranking of carbohydrate foods based on how they affect the body's blood glucose level. Individual foods are compared to white bread or glucose. High GI foods produce a greater increase in blood glucose levels than low GI foods.

Grams of Total Carbohydrate vs. Grams of Sugar

Managing your blood sugar level is important not only for people with diabetes but for anyone trying to lose weight or maintain a healthy weight. This is especially true following weight loss surgery. But it isn't just eating sugar that raises your blood sugar level; all carbohydrates break down in the body as glucose (sugar) when digested and absorbed. A carb ... is a carb ... is a carb.

Carbohydrates include a variety of foods – everything from salad greens to chocolate cake! Your body doesn't know the difference between a donut or a whole-wheat bagel, a glass of orange juice or a glass of soda. The orange juice and the whole-wheat bagel would provide more nutrition, such as fiber, vitamin C and potassium, than the soda or the donut, but *all* of these foods would raise your blood sugar. Even "no sugar added" foods, such as fruit, vegetables, "all natural" fruit juice, unsweetened cereal, whole grain bread and sugar-free cookies will cause your blood sugar to rise because all these foods are rich in total carbohydrate and *all* carbohydrates turn into sugar in the body.

But before you go labeling carbohydrates as "bad" foods, let me assure you that these foods are an essential part of a healthy diet. However, the amount of carbohydrate in your diet can make the difference between gaining and losing weight. Many people associate the dumping syndrome with sugar from sweets, but fail to consider other carbohydrate-rich foods. As we will discuss in Chapter 22, learning to count the grams of total carbohydrate from each food, not just the grams of sugar, is important to prevent the dumping syndrome and to maximize weight loss. When you eat more than the recommended number of carbohydrate grams at one sitting, regardless of the nutrition content of the food, you are at risk for dumping. Period.

Following this plan, you will still enjoy a variety of carbohydrates, but in more modest amounts than you may be accustomed to. About a third of your calories during the day will come from this nutrient. You will learn to balance your total carbohydrate intake at each meal between low carbohydrate foods, like non-starchy vegetables, and higher carbohydrate foods such as fruit, bread, pasta and starchy vegetables. When you understand carbohydrate counting and what your "budget" for total carbohydrate is at each meal, you will see how to include all foods in your diet and still reach your goal weight. We will discuss specific guidelines for balancing carbohydrate, protein and fat in Chapter 24. (See Table 21.1 for a sample meal including carbohydrate-rich foods within appropriate guidelines).

Glycemic Index

There seems to be a lot of confusion about carbohydrates even among health practitioners. In a recently released book for bariatric patients I read the following recommendation: "...Instead of having a serving of pineapple (which is high in calories and sugar,) have a serving of strawberries." This implies that some fruits are "good" and some are "bad" which is simply *not* true and is very misleading!

Table 21.1
Considering the Grams of Total Carbohydrates Per Meal Using the Maintenance Diet Recommendations of Limiting Total Carbohydrate to 20-30 grams per Meal

Sample Meal:
½ ham & cheese sandwich
a piece of fruit
a handful of pretzels.

The combined carbohydrate content from the bread (10 grams per slice), fruit (15 grams per serving) and pretzels (12 grams per serving) would be too high (37 grams total.) However, the bread plus the fruit (25 grams) OR the bread plus the pretzels (22 grams) would keep the carbohydrate content for this meal within the recommended maintenance diet level of 20-30 grams per meal.

Some carbohydrates raise the level of sugar in your blood stream faster and higher than others. This can be demonstrated by a measure known as the glycemic index (GI) of a food. Pure glucose is used as a reference and is given a value of 100, meaning that it causes a very rapid rise in blood glucose. Other carbohydrates are ranked relative to glucose and are given specific values, with a value of 70 or higher considered to be high and a value of 55 or lower considered low (see Table 21.2.).

A high GI food when eaten as part of a meal that contains protein, fiber, fat or acid (e.g. vinegar or lemon juice) will become a lower GI food. For example, when you eat a baked potato (a high GI food) with steak (high protein and fat) the GI of the potato is lower. That's because the protein and fat in the steak will slow down the rate at which the whole meal is digested and absorbed which results in a slower rise in blood sugar.

Table 21.2
The Glycemic Index of White Bread vs. Legumes

Example: white rice or white bread eaten alone would have a similar effect on your blood sugar as glucose.

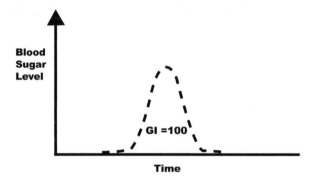

(**GI = 100:** the greatest rise in blood sugar.)

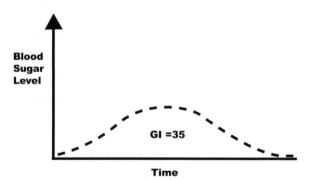

Higher fiber foods, like legumes, take longer to digest and absorb. Thus, legumes have a lower glycemic index (**GI = 35**); meaning they would elevate the blood sugar slower & lower overall than foods with a higher GI.

GI does not indicate whether a food is "good" or "bad." It simply measures the affect of a food or meal on the body's blood glucose level. For example, rice cakes and instant oatmeal have a high GI, whereas pound cake and chocolate éclairs (because of their fat content) are relatively low.

You should be raising an eyebrow if using the GI to make food choices leads you to label strawberries as "good" and pineapple as "bad," or to avoid bananas, carrots and oatmeal because they have a high GI and choose pound cake with a lower GI. A wide range of fruits, vegetables, beans and whole grains should be included in your diet in moderation. If you eat a large portion of any carbohydrate-rich food you are at risk for dumping. GI may be useful for determining if you will experience early or late dumping; but do you really care if you dump now or later? Or would you rather prevent dumping altogether?

> *You may notice that certain carbohydrates affect you differently than others. Some people find that eating pasta or rice makes them feel bloated and uncomfortable. Others report feeling hungry sooner after eating simple carbohydrates like white bread or sweets. Pay attention to the way you feel after eating to find the foods that make you feel your best.*

Bottom Line: There are no good foods or bad foods. As we will discuss in the chapters to follow, your best approach at every meal is to choose a protein-rich food first; then fill your plate around that with controlled portions of total carbohydrate (see Table 24.1 and 25.2.). You will find applying the GI of various foods is not as important as simply balancing your protein-rich foods with the total grams of carbohydrate at each meal. To optimize health and weight management include a variety of nutrient-dense carbohydrates such as fruit, vegetables and whole grains. And please, go easy on the pound cake!

What About Net Carbs?

"Net carbs" or "low-impact carbs" refers to the carbohydrate content of a food after subtracting the grams of sugar alcohol and fiber. Just a few years ago, none of us had ever heard of the term "net carbs" because food manufacturers were simply omitting fiber and sugar alcohol grams from the nutrition-facts label to make the total carbohydrate content appear low. This was very misleading for consumers, (and even dangerous for people with health conditions, such as diabetes, which requires good blood sugar control) because it made food products appear to be much lower in carbohydrate than they actually were. The FDA now requires that *all sources of* carbohydrate be included in the count of total carbohydrate grams.

Foods that have a larger percentage of total carbohydrate in the form of sugar alcohol and/or fiber will have a lower glycemic index because these forms of carbohydrate are digested and absorbed more *slowly* (or not at all, in the case of insoluble fiber.) However, the GI of a food may determine *when* you dump, but it is the total grams of carbohydrate that determines *if* you dump.

Bottom Line: "net carbs" does not mean "free carbs." Count the grams of total carbohydrate from all foods eaten per meal and stay within the guidelines for carbohydrate intake per meal (see Table 24.1.)

Sugar Alcohols

Don't let the name fool you. Sugar alcohol does not contain ethanol, which is the kind of alcohol found in beer, wine, and liquor. However, these ingredients were given the consumer friendly name "sugar alcohol" because part of their chemical structure resembles sugar and part resembles alcohol.

Sugar alcohols occur naturally in plant foods such as fruits and berries. They are used as sweeteners and bulking agents in foods and provide about 2.6 calories per gram compared to 4 calories per gram of regular sugar. Sugar alcohol is absorbed more slowly than sugar, which prevents your blood sugar and insulin levels from spiking. Products sweetened with sugar alcohols may provide some lower carbohydrate alternatives to post-op patients. But beware! Many of these products still contain significant amounts of total carbohydrate.

> *Sugar alcohols provide about 2.6 calories per gram compared to 4 calories per gram of regular sugar. But beware! Many of these products still contain significant amounts of total carbohydrate.*

Bottom Line: Foods sweetened with sugar alcohols often still contain significant amounts of carbohydrate. It is important to check the food label for grams of total carbohydrate to minimize the risk of dumping and enhance overall weight loss.

Sugar Alcohols vs. Artificial Sweeteners

Sugar alcohols and artificial sweeteners, such as saccharin (Sweet & Low ™), aspartame (Equal™ or NutraSweet™), and sucralose (Splenda™) are not one and the same. First, sugar alcohols contain carbohydrate so they will cause a rise in blood sugar. Artificial sweeteners will not affect blood sugar because they do not contain any carbohydrate. Second, sugar alcohols contain an average of 2.6 calories per gram while artificial sweeteners contain 0 calories. Both sugar substitutes can be useful for weight management (and diabetes management) when used properly. See Appendix E for a comparison of sugar substitutes.

Table 21.3
The Pros and Cons of Sugar Alcohols

Pros
- Contain fewer calories
- Do not promote tooth decay
- Add texture to food
- Retain moisture in foods
- Prevent foods from browning when heated

Cons
- Bloating and diarrhea are common side effects.
- Large doses may have a laxative effect often misinterpreted as dumping.
- Consumers commonly mistake foods containing sugar alcohols to be "calorie-free" or low calorie foods.
- Regular intake of these food products may increase calorie intake overall leading to weight gain.

Fiber

What your mom might have called "roughage," dietitians know as fiber. Fiber is a type of carbohydrate found in plants. Because the body cannot digest and absorb it, fiber itself does not provide any calories. Therefore, high fiber foods that are low in fat, such as fruits and vegetables, are low in calories.

Although fiber is not considered an essential nutrient, the U.S. Surgeon General and many health organizations recommend a diet containing 20-35 grams of fiber per day. By including just 7-10 grams of fiber per meal, as part of your 20-30 grams of total carbohydrate, you can meet the dietary guidelines for fiber and enhance your post-op diet lifestyle.

Table 21.4
Fiber-Rich Foods

Food	Grams of Fiber
Broccoli, ¾ Cup, cooked	7.0
Dried Figs, 2	7.0
Lentils, 1/3 Cup, raw	5.5
3 Tbsp. All-Bran Cereal	5.0
Baked beans, 1/3 Cup	5.3
Artichokes, 4 small hearts	4.0
Triscuits, 4 crackers	4.0
Spinach, 1 Cup, raw	3.5
Carrots, ½ Cup, cooked	3.4
Apple, 1 small	3.0
Banana, 1 medium	3.0
Nature's Own White Wheat Bread, 1 slice	3.0
Beets, ½ Cup, cooked	2.5
Peach, 1 medium	2.3
Dried Apricots, 2 halves	2.0
Celery, ¼ Cup, raw	2.0
Olives, 6 green or black	1.2

Post-Chapter Exercises:

+ *Exercise One:* Practice reading food labels and using the dietary exchanges in Appendix B and C for tallying your grams of total carbohydrate at each meal. If you were used to counting grams of sugar in the past, practice re-training your eye to look for grams of total carbohydrate.

- *Exercise Two:* Remember products that boast low levels of "net carbs" or "impact carbs" may be helpful in finding some foods with a lower amount of total carbohydrate. But be sure you always check the nutrition facts label and count the grams of total carbohydrate toward your meal budget.
- *Exercise Three:* If you eat and drink a lot of sugar-free products containing sugar alcohols, remember a side effect in some people can be gas, bloating and diarrhea. Don't assume that it is dumping. Keep a food diary and track what you are eating; experiment with decreasing your intake of sugar alcohol and note if symptoms improve.
- *Exercise Four:* Identify several carbohydrate foods you like that contain 5 grams or more of fiber per serving. Plan to include these foods at meals in place of lower fiber carbohydrates.

Twenty-two

WHAT YOU NEED TO KNOW ABOUT DUMPING

In This Chapter
- Understand the physiology of the dumping syndrome and how to prevent it.
- Recognize symptoms associated with early and late dumping.
- Identify that total carbohydrates, not just sugar, play a role in the dumping syndrome.

Key Words to Know
- *reactive hypoglycemia:* a drop in blood sugar caused by insulin secretion following a high carbohydrate intake.

What is Dumping?

Most of you have heard the stories, and probably have a few of your own to tell, but do you really understand what dumping is? In my practice I have seen a lot of misconceptions about the dumping syndrome. One phrase I hear most often during consults with patients gaining weight after surgery is, "I don't have dumping ... I never throw up!" This is a dangerous misconception to have because dumping is one of the most common reasons for weight loss plateaus and weight re-gain following surgery. Yet dumping rarely involves vomiting. So what exactly is dumping?

The dumping syndrome refers to the rapid passage of food from your stomach pouch into the small intestine. This causes a shift of fluid from the blood plasma to rush into the intestines where the lump of food you ate now sits. You might experience sweating, dizziness, lightheadedness, nausea, diarrhea, rapid heart beat, low blood pressure, cramping, weakness and/or headache. These symptoms may occur in *any combination or not at all.*

So you see, you may *feel* nauseated when dumping, but because the food is rapidly moving in the opposite direction, you are more likely to experience diarrhea than vomiting. (See Chapter 29 for more on vomiting)

Early Dumping

Early dumping is typically associated with a quick onset of symptoms immediately after eating a meal that is low in protein and high in simple carbohydrates like sugar, white bread, or white rice. As a result, fluid is drawn from blood plasma into your small intestine. This fluid shift is the body's attempt to dilute the concentrated food that has just been dumped there. Symptoms may include abdominal pain, bloating, diarrhea, nausea, cramping and fullness. Symptoms typically improve when you are lying down and tend to pass within 30-60 minutes.

Late Dumping

Late dumping typically occurs 1-3 hours after a meal that is high in total carbohydrate. Symptoms are a result of the fluid shift from your blood to your small intestine, which ultimately decreases the amount of blood circulating in your body and decreases cardiac output. Symptoms are more neurological in nature, and include weakness, shakiness, feeling lightheaded or dizzy, rapid heartbeat and cold sweat.

Delayed dumping is also known as *reactive hypoglycemia*. This means that the body responds to a rapid rise in blood sugar by stimulating the pancreas to secrete insulin. This high insulin level is responsible for the big drop in blood sugar that follows. Thus, the symptoms of late dumping are similar to those of a low blood sugar, but sugar is the last thing you need! Treatment for the condition includes a protein and carbohydrate-rich snack, such as cheese with fruit or a glass of low-fat milk.

Keep in mind that many patients experience such subtle symptoms after eating carbohydrate-rich foods they do not realize they have dumped. This is a problem because dumping leaves your stomach empty, causing you to feel hunger shortly after meals. Over time, this leads to weight gain if hunger causes you to eat more calories from frequent snacks and larger meals. Patients tend to have a "love-hate" relationship with dumping. Those who have a strong dumping response are often times more compliant with diet recommendations and more successful with weight loss overall because of the negative re-enforcement. However, nobody likes to dump.

Bottom Line: Any *combination* of food with a high amount of *total carbohydrate* will result in dumping. Regular meals containing protein and complex carbohydrates will decrease the risk of early and late dumping. If you experience frequent hunger at any point following surgery, keep in mind that it may be due to dumping, even if hunger is your *only* symptom. Contact your registered dietitian right away before you start re-gaining weight. (See Appendix F and visit our web site at www. theroadtowlssuccess.com for a series of sample meals with appropriate combinations of protein and carbohydrate-rich foods.)

Post-Chapter Exercises:

- ◆ *Exercise One:* Keep a food diary this week and make note of how you feel immediately and several hours after eating a meal. If you experience any symptoms of dumping, reflect on your food choices and note any changes you could have made.
- ◆ *Exercise Two:* Keep quick protein-rich foods on hand like pop-top or zip-top pouches of water packed tuna, salmon or chicken, peanut butter, deli-meats, string cheese, hard boiled eggs (boil a dozen and then refrigerate), a can of nuts (any variety) and protein bars (see Appendix G for a list of protein-rich snack bars appropriate for the pot-op diet; see Table 23.2 and 26.4 for ideas of protein-rich foods and snacks.)

Twenty-three

GOT PROTEIN?

In This Chapter
- Understand the role protein plays in maximizing your weight loss and weight-loss maintenance.
- Calculate your daily protein needs.
- Identify the amount of protein in food.

Key Words to Know
- *Ideal body weight:* An estimation of appropriate body weight for health based on your height and frame size.

Protein

Protein is a critical part of your daily diet following surgery because of its role in repairing and building cell tissue. Protein is essential for promoting healing after surgery, keeping your immune system strong and preserving your muscle mass. I have observed less nausea, less hair loss, improved weight loss and fewer complications in general with patients who consistently meet the initial protein goal of 60 grams daily. There are fewer negative symptoms if the maintenance diet goal of 60-100 grams of protein daily (or about 1.0 - 1.2 grams of protein per kg of ideal body weight) is met. * This goal can easily be reached by including solid, protein-rich foods such as beef, pork, poultry, fish, eggs, legumes, cheese, yogurt, nuts and seeds at every meal.

> ***Eating appropriate protein at each meal minimizes your risk
> of dumping, and keeps you satisfied between meals, so you are
> less likely to snack or over-eat later in the day. Meeting your
> protein goal at each meal also decreases the risk of frequent
> weight- loss plateaus or re-gaining weight.***

Each protein-rich food has its own sequence of amino acids, the
building blocks of protein. So it's important to regularly include a variety
of protein-rich foods in the diet. However, not all protein-rich foods have
the same number of calories because the fat and water content vary.

Table 23.1
**Calculating Daily Protein Needs Based on Height,
Frame Size and Ideal Body Weight**

Step One: Calculate Ideal Body Weight
Ideal weight for height for women is determined by starting
with 100# for the first 5 feet and adding or subtracting 5
pounds for each inch of height above or below 5 feet. Add 10%
to ideal body weight for medium to large frame sizes. A 5'4"
woman with a medium frame would have an ideal body weight
range of 120-132# calculated by: (100# + (4"x 5#) + 10%.)

Ideal weight for men is determined by starting with 106# for the
first 5 feet and adding 6 pounds for each additional inch of height
above 5 feet. A 6'0" foot male would have an ideal body weight
range of 178-196# calculated by: (106# + (12" X 6#) +10%.)

Step Two: Calculating Daily Protein Needs
To estimate your minimum protein requirement take your ideal
weight for height calculated in Step 1 and divide it by 2.2 to get
your ideal weight for height in kilograms (kg). Multiply that
number by 1.0 and 1.2 grams of protein to estimate your
daily protein goal. Example: a 5'8" woman would have an
ideal body weight of 140-154#; divide these two weights by
2.2 to get 64 - 70 kg; now multiply these two numbers by 1.0
and 1.2 to get a goal range of 64 - 84 grams of protein/day.

Cheese, nuts, and peanut butter are good examples of protein-rich foods that are also high in fat. Yes, you can get a good dose of protein from your favorite cheese, nuts and nut-butters, but you also get more calories because these foods are higher in fat. Most cheeses have 100 calories per ounce, while fish or baked chicken has about 30 calories per ounce.

Bottom line: calories count, but variety is important. Include a variety of protein-rich foods in your diet on a regular basis, but keep an eye on the fat.

A Natural Appetite Suppressant

Protein-rich foods can be thought of as natural appetite suppressants because they take longer than carbohydrate to digest and absorb, and they are least likely to cause dumping. This means you will sense feeling full with smaller portions of food and for longer periods of time when eating protein-rich foods.

Balance protein with carbohydrate and fat instead of eating a high carbohydrate meal with little or no protein. Breakfast is a great example of this. Patients often tell me that they are hungrier on the days they eat breakfast than on the days they skip it.

"What do you have for breakfast?" I always ask. Inevitably, the answer will be high carbohydrate foods without a good protein source, such as toast with jelly, toaster pastries, or cereal and milk. When we add protein to the mix, appetite control improves and weight loss soon follows.

Making Room for Protein

Protein should always be eaten first at a meal. This ensures the daily goal for protein is met and maximizes weight loss overall. By eating protein-rich foods first, you are more likely to "crowd out" excess calories from carbohydrate and fat rather than making them the primary focus of the meal. A good guideline for protein intake once you have reached your maintenance diet is 3-4 oz. or 21-28 grams of protein at each meal. (See Table 23.1 to calculate your protein needs based on your height, frame size and ideal body weight.)

Table 23.2
Examples of Protein-Rich Foods

Serving Size	Grams of Protein	Grams of Carbohydrate
3 oz. Chicken Breast	21.0	0
3 Slices of Bacon	10.0	0.5
3 oz. Lean Pot Roast	25.0	0
3 oz. Lean Ground Beef	22.0	0
3 oz. Roasted Turkey, White	25.0	0
3 X 1 oz. Slices Deli Turkey	21.0	0
3 oz. Roasted Deer Meat	25.0	0
3 oz. Grilled Tuna	23.0	0
4 Large Clams (9 small)	11.0	2.2
6 Medium Oysters	5.9	3.3
3 oz. Salmon	21.0	0
15 Large Shrimp	18.0	0
1 Large Egg	7.0	0.5
1 oz. Cheddar Cheese	7.1	0.4
½ Cup 1% Cottage Cheese	16.0	3.0
2 Tablespoons Peanut Butter	8.5	6.0
¼ Cup Almonds	7.0	7.0
Veggie Burger (1 patty)	11.2	8.9
6 oz. Light Fruit Flavor Yogurt	5.0	16.0

Reading food labels and using resources like Table 4.2 may be useful as you begin learning more about including protein-rich foods at each meal. However, keep in mind that some general guidelines can make tallying up your protein as easy as looking at your plate of food. For example, an ounce of cheese, 1 slice of deli meat or 1 large egg has about 1 serving or 7 grams of protein. A 3 oz. piece of meat is equivalent to a deck of cards or about a "palm-size" portion. Once you reach your maintenance diet, you should include a *minimum* of 3 oz. (or 21 grams) of protein at each of your three meals daily. Depending on your activity level, daily calorie needs and your individual pouch size, you may be eating more protein than this per meal. We will practice using visual cues for portion control in chapter 25.

Post-Chapter Exercises:

- *Exercise One:* Using your ideal body weight for height, calculate your minimum daily protein goal.
- *Exercise Two:* If you are experiencing hunger between meals, be sure you are eating a minimum of 21 grams of protein from a solid food source at each meal.
- *Exercise Three:* Choose 3 new protein-rich foods you have not tried or just haven't eaten in a while and include them in your meal planning this week.
- *Exercise Four:* Try a new recipe this week for a protein-rich entrée. See Appendix F and visit our web site at www.theroadtowlssuccess.com for some ideas.

Twenty-four

YOUR OWNER'S MANUAL: 6 STEPS TO SUCCESS

In This Chapter
- Understand that weight re-gain is possible after surgery.
- Identify specific dietary budgets for eating protein, carbohydrate and fat at each meal.
- Understand why fluids should be consumed separate from meals.
- Identify appropriate beverage choices.
- Learn strategies for avoiding hunger between meals.
- Recognize the bariatric food guide pyramid.
- Identify the six keys to life-long weight loss success.

Key Words to Know
- *grazing:* eating small, frequent meals throughout the day.

Put on Your Tool Belt

You may have heard the expression, "weight loss surgery is only a tool." This is so true! There is nothing magical about losing weight after gastric bypass surgery. Patients often act surprised when I tell them, "It is possible to re-gain some or all of your weight after this surgery." Unfortunately, I meet patients on a regular basis who have re-gained a portion or all of their weight; however, these are typically patients who never learned how to use their weight-loss tool.

The small stomach pouch created by your surgeon is your "weight loss tool." Successful weight loss depends on your understanding of how to use that tool. Although most people will successfully lose weight the first year or two following surgery, this is primarily a result of taking in fewer calories. The real question is, will you reach your goal weight, and maintain it as your weight loss slows and your hunger level increases? The guidelines discussed in this chapter will help you understand the keys to long-term weight loss success.

Table 24.1
Your Owner's Manual - 6 Steps to Success

1. Always choose a **protein-rich** food *first* and include a *minimum* of 21-28 grams of protein per meal.
2. Budget your **total carbohydrate** intake to *20-30 grams per meal*.
3. Limit your **fat** intake to 10-15 grams per meal.
4. **Do not graze on foods** throughout the day. Eat 3 regular meals.
5. **Do not *drink* your calories OR drink with meals.** Drink only calorie-free, non-carbonated fluids *in between* meals; and be sure to get 64 oz. daily.
6. **Exercise** regularly to help reach and maintain your goal weight. Be sure to include both aerobic and resistance training (See Chapter 31 for exercise guidelines and sample programs.)

Owner's Manual Step One

Choose a protein-rich food *first* every time you eat. Protein-rich foods take longer to digest than carbohydrate. This means when you eat protein-rich foods you are likely to stay full for a longer period of time, supporting your goal to eat fewer calories each day. A good goal is to eat a minimum of 3-4 oz. or 21-28 grams of protein per meal, 3 times per day.

Owner's Manual Step Two

Carbohydrate-rich foods are an important part of a healthy diet. However, too much carbohydrate at meals will cause dumping and leave you hungry between meals. A good guideline is to limit total carbohydrate to 20-30 grams per meal, 3 times a day. It is my experience that most people do well averaging an intake at the upper level recommended here (30 grams of total carbohydrate per meal) by 1-2 years following surgery and beyond. Keep in mind that specific dietary needs may vary based on the individual and/or any changes in physical activity.

Owner's Manual Step Three

Fat, like protein, slows the rate at which your body will digest a meal. However, at 9 calories per gram of fat, it is easy to consume excess calories if you eat a large proportion of your calories from fat. You may also experience dumping-type symptoms after eating a very high-fat meal. Limit fat to 10-15 grams per meal. For heart health, remember to choose monounsaturated and polyunsaturated fats the majority of the time.

> *Your maintenance diet should consist of about 1 to 1 and ½ cups of food per meal 3 times a day.*

Owner's Manual Step Four

Immediately following surgery you will have swelling in your stomach pouch, and your appetite will be low. When you begin adding solid foods back to the diet, your portion sizes will be just 2-4 tablespoons at each meal. Many surgeons and dietitians recommend eating several small meals throughout the day during this stage to ensure adequate nutrition. Between 3 to 6 months post-op you will be able to accommodate larger portion sizes. At this point you should discontinue eating little meals throughout the day and focus on eating 3 regular meals daily. By eating little meals, or "grazing," throughout the day you will never quite feel full. This leaves you vulnerable to eating more frequently and taking in too many total carbohydrates and calories.

Eating just 3 meals daily will increase feelings of fullness following meals and enhance overall weight loss. Your maintenance diet should consist of about 1 to 1 ½ cups of food per meal 3 times a day.

Owner's Manual Step Five

Initially after surgery it will be difficult to eat or drink much at one time because post-operative swelling reduces the size of your pouch. To avoid uncomfortable complications, get in the habit of drinking fluids between meals throughout the day. Do not drink at mealtime.

As the stomach pouch heals and swelling subsides, you will be able to hold larger volumes of fluid and food. However, it is still important to separate your liquids and solids. Combining fluids with your food at mealtime may cause you to feel full sooner, thus limiting the amount of protein and nutrition you are able to consume at that meal. However, this sensation of fullness will be followed by a rapid return of hunger. Because when food is eaten along with fluids, the meal empties the pouch much faster, leaving you hungry. This leads to weight-loss plateaus and weight re-gain from a higher calorie intake overall.

Bottom Line: stop drinking fluids about 15 to 30 minutes before a meal, and wait 60-90 minutes after eating before drinking again. To avoid dehydration and encourage satiation between meals, plan ahead by sipping on fluids in between meals throughout the day. Drinking fluids between meals gives you a feeling of fullness until it is time to eat your next meal. Aim for 64 oz. of calorie-free, non-carbonated fluids every day.

Minimize high calorie beverages

Meal replacement drinks, milk, fruit juice, soup, or any fluid with calories is ***not*** a good choice after surgery. That's because liquids pass through your small stomach pouch very quickly. Thus high calorie liquids do nothing to satisfy your hunger, yet they contribute excess calories to your daily intake. This encourages weight gain.

> *Weight loss surgery is a tool. Your success depends on how well you use that tool.*

You may understand this guideline better when you consider that the first thing I would recommend to someone who has lost too much weight following surgery would be to add meal replacement drinks or other liquid calories between or during meals. Why? Because high calorie fluids will increase the amount of calories consumed, but will not decrease the person's appetite. However, if we tried to get the person's calorie level up by adding a steak in between meals, their appetite would decrease and they would not be able to eat enough to gain weight.

Questions to Ask if You Feel Hungry In Between Meals:

1. Did I include a solid, protein-rich food at my last meal? (goal: a minimum of 21 grams per meal)
2. Did I meet, but not exceed, my budget for total carbohydrate? (goal: 20-30 grams per meal)
3. Did I eat enough food at my last meal? (goal: a minimum of 300-400 calories)
4. Did I stop drinking 15-30 minutes before starting my last meal?
5. Did I wait 60-90 minutes before resuming fluids after my last meal?
6. Have I been drinking enough fluids today or could my hunger actually be a sign of dehydration? (See chapter 29 for more on dehydration.)

Bottom Line: do not drink your calories. Get your protein from solid-food sources and drink plenty of water and other sugar-free, non-carbonated drinks in between meals. There are a lot of new beverages showing up on grocery store shelves that would be appropriate choices. When in doubt check the nutrition facts food label. If a beverage is non-carbonated and has zero grams of total carbohydrate it's a good choice.

Try some of these non-carbonated, calorie free drinks	
Beverage	*Grams of Carbohydrate Per Serving*
Crystal Light™	0 grams
Fruit20 Water™	0 grams
Sugar-Free Kool-Aid™,	0 grams
Tang™, Wylers™, Country Time™	0 grams
Propel Water™	2 grams
Minute Maid Light™	2 grams

Owner's Manual Step Six

Exercise is an important component of your post-op lifestyle to improve weight loss, body composition and weight loss maintenance. See Chapter 31 for more information on the basic components of fitness and a list of sample exercise programs.

Post-Chapter Exercises:

- ◆ *Exercise One:* Practice building some meals with a minimum of 21 grams of protein and no more than 25-30 grams of carbohydrate.
- ◆ *Exercise Two:* Try a few new beverages this week to add variety and minimize the temptation to choose a carbonated or high sugar drink. Be sure to read the food label and choose beverages with zero grams of total carbohydrate.
- ◆ *Exercise Three:* Use a stop watch one day this week to get a realistic idea of how long you are waiting after meals before you drink. Check if you are waiting long enough between stopping fluids and starting a meal.
- ◆ *Exercise Four:* This week, plan your meals the day before to support your goal to eat 3 regular meals daily; do not skip meals!

Twenty-five

KEEPING IT SIMPLE: YOUR EATING PLAN IS AS EASY AS 1, 2, 3

In This Chapter
- Learn the plate method approach to building post-op meals.
- Learn to reference the dietary exchange lists for choosing appropriate portion sizes.
- Identify portion sizes visually using common objects.

The Plate Method

The guidelines discussed in the last chapter gave you the basic framework for balancing carbohydrate, protein and fat. In this chapter we'll practice a visual approach to meal building, which I call "the plate method." As you will see in Table 25.2, the plate method makes creating post-op meals as easy as 1, 2, 3!

With the plate method, foods are divided into three sections. To put together a meal all you have to do is pick one food from each category. The foods and portions listed are designed to add up to meals of approximately 300-400 calories. Initially you might want to weigh or measure out the various serving sizes listed in each category. The idea behind the plate method is to simplify meal building by giving you a visual reference for making accurate estimates of portion sizes. I've also found that associating a common object with the recommended portion size of a food helps people better plan the amount of food they are going to eat. See Table 25.1 for some common memory aids for gauging portion sizes. Then try creating a few of your own as you practice building some meals applying the plate method.

Table 25.1
Objects Commonly Associated with Food Portions

Food	*Approximate Size*
3-4 oz. of meat	a deck of cards or the palm of your hand
1 oz. of meat or cheese	a domino
1 serving of fruit	a tennis ball
1 Cup cooked vegetables	a baseball

Guidelines for Building a Meal

Follow these three steps to practice creating some meals using the plate method. Balancing your favorite foods this way will decrease your risk of dumping, early return of hunger, frequent hunger, weight loss plateaus and/or weight gain.

1) Choose your **protein first** at every meal. Ensure a minimum of three ounces or twenty-one grams of protein per meal. This would be about the size of a deck of cards or the palm of your hand. (See Table 25.3 and Appendix A.)
2) Choose a **low carbohydrate vegetable second** to increase satiation without loading up on carbohydrates. (See table 25.4 and Appendix B) Remember one-half cup of non-starchy vegetables (cooked) and 1 cup (raw) has just five grams of carbohydrate. A half-cup is approximately the size of a tennis ball; one cup is about the size of a baseball.
3) Choose high carbohydrate foods like fruit, starchy vegetables, breads, rice and pasta last to avoid filling up on these foods and crowding out your protein and low carbohydrate foods. One high carbohydrate serving is equivalent to fifteen grams of carbohydrate. (See Table 25.5 and Appendix C.)

Table 25.2

The Plate Method
Building Your Post-Op Meals is as Easy as 1...2...3!!!

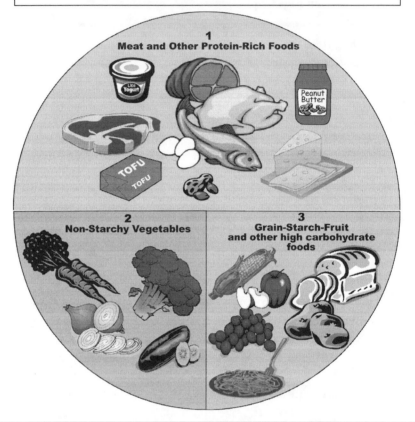

Plate Section 1 + (See Table 25.3 *and* Appendix A)	Plate Section 2 + (See Table 25.4 *and* Appendix B)	Plate Section 3 (See Table 25.5 *and* Appendix C)
2 Eggs + 1 oz. Cheese	½ Cup Red Pepper	1 Banana, medium
2 Eggs + 3 Slices Bacon	½ Cup Sliced Tomatoes	1 ¼ Cup Strawberries
2 oz. turkey + 1 oz. Cheese	Lettuce and Tomato	2 Slices of Bread
3-4 oz. Chicken Breast	1 Cup Green Beans	2/3 Cup Corn
3 oz. Shrimp	1 Cup Salad Greens	10-15 French Fries

Table 25.3
Section 1: Choose your protein first
　　One serving of protein is equivalent to seven grams of protein or one ounce of meat. *The examples below are combinations of protein-rich foods that meet the minimum plate method goal of three ounces or twenty one grams of protein per meal.* Use the dietary exchanges for protein listed in Appendix A to create more meal combinations of your own.

Examples of 3 oz. or 21 grams of protein:
3 eggs or ¾ Cup of egg replacement
2 eggs + 1 oz. of cheese
1 egg + 1 oz. of cheese + 2-3 slices of bacon
3-4 oz. of meat or fish
15 large shrimp
2 slices of deli meat + 1 oz. of cheese
6 oz. of light yogurt + 2 oz. of cheese
½ Cup low-fat cottage cheese + ¼ Cup almonds

Table 25.4
Section 2: Non-Starchy Vegetables
See Appendix B for a complete list of non-starchy, low carbohydrate vegetables.

Food
1/2 Cup broccoli, *cooked*
1/2 Cup cauliflower, *cooked*
1/2 Cup collards, *cooked*
1/2 Cup green beans, *cooked*
1 Cup salad greens

Table 25.5
Section 3: High Carbohydrate Foods Such as Fruit, Starchy Vegetables, Bread, Rice and Pasta
See Appendix C for a complete list of high carbohydrate foods. The examples shown here represent one serving or fifteen grams of carbohydrate.

Food	1 Serving = 15 grams of Carbohydrate
Banana, medium	1/2
Blueberries	3/4 Cup
Bread	1 slice
Grapes, small	17
English Muffin	1/2
Rice, white or brown	1/3 Cup
Spaghetti, cooked	1/2 Cup

When you add 1 serving from section 3 to 1 serving from section 2 (5 grams) you will meet the low end of your carbohydrate budget of 20 grams per meal. Feel free to be creative with your meals by combining different types of food from the same category. Also, remember to increase the number of servings in Section 2 and/or 3 (up to 30 grams of carbohydrate per meal) as your calorie needs increase.

Post-Chapter Exercises:

- *Exercise One:* Practice using the "plate method" approach to creating meals. The more you practice using visual cues to balance your protein, carbohydrate and fat, the less you will have to rely on reading labels, dietary exchange lists and food scales.
- *Exercise Two:* Change your mind-set if you are used to thinking of foods as "good" or "bad." Carbohydrates are essential and eating too few can sabotage your weight loss goals. Plan to include 20-30 grams of carbohydrate per meal.
- *Exercise Three:* Plan ahead, and keep protein-rich snacks on-hand. Stock the refrigerator at work and home with snack-size yogurt, string cheese and deli meat. Stash a can of nuts in your desk drawer. Keep a protein bar in your glove box or purse.

Twenty-six

DOING THE MATH – THE NUMBERS JUST DON'T ADD UP!

In This Chapter
- Understand the calculations for determining the amount of carbohydrate, fat and protein at each meal.
- Understand why diets that severely restrict carbohydrates aren't realistic or healthy.
- Compare the guidelines from your owner's manual with the Institute of Medicine's dietary guidelines.
- Recognize when snacking between meals is appropriate and how to make good snack choices.

Considering Calories

As discussed earlier, by 3 to 6 months following surgery you will notice being able to hold more food in your stomach pouch at one sitting. During this time you should transition toward eating 3 regular meals daily and discontinue eating between meals. Between 6 to 12 months post-op you will be eating about 900 to 1,200 calories per day or 300 to 400 calories per meal. It is best to keep your daily intake within this range until you have reached your goal weight and are maintaining it there comfortably. Keep in mind that your calorie needs vary as your activity level increases or decreases and everybody's metabolism is different.

If you experience frequent hunger accompanied by weight loss that your surgeon feels is too rapid or too slow, you might need to adjust your calories. Consult with a registered dietitian to assess your diet, rule out dumping and take the guesswork out of planning appropriate diet changes. (See the guidelines discussed in Chapter 29 should you begin losing weight *below* your goal weight.)

Doing the Math

Many fad diets for post-op patients continue to emphasize a *very low* carbohydrate, low fat diet. Some go as far as recommending a severe carbohydrate restriction of 25 grams per day. However, as you are about to see, these numbers just don't add up!

Every gram of fat has 9 calories. Compare that to the 4 calories in every gram of carbohydrate or protein, and you can see why fat gets a bad rap. You're getting more than twice the calories for every gram of fat you eat than you would get from a gram of carbohydrate or protein. However, as we discussed in chapter twenty, fat is an essential part of the diet. An appropriate calorie range for fat, using the guidelines from your owner's manual, would be 10-15 grams or 90 – 135 fat calories per meal (10-15 grams of fat multiplied by 9 calories per gram.)

Table 26.1

Calculating Calories from Carbohydrate

There are 4 calories per gram of carbohydrate. If you ate just 25 grams of carbohydrate per day: 25 grams of carbohydrate X 4 calories per gram = 100 carbohydrate calories per day. Divide 100 calories by 3 meals to get 33 calories per meal from carbohydrate or just 100 of your 900-1200 calories per day from carbohydrate. **This is too low!**

If you followed fad guidelines to limit your carbohydrates to 25 grams per day, that would allow for a mere 33 calories or 8.25 grams of carbohydrate per meal (see Table 26.1.) This would be equivalent to 1 tbsp. of raisins or 2 tbsp. of grits; this is too low!

Remember, the average calorie range for your maintenance diet is 300-400 calories per meal. But, what do you have left to eat? You guessed it … protein! The problem is you have a little *too much* protein. Subtracting your calories from carbohydrate and fat, you are left with 132-277 protein calories (300 - 400 calories minus 33 carbohydrate calories minus 90 – 135 fat calories). This is the equivalent of 5 to 10 oz. of meat per meal! It would not be physically comfortable or *possible* to eat this much protein in one sitting. Not to mention excluding nutrient-dense carbohydrates such as fruit, vegetables and whole grains to make room for excessive protein does not make a lot of sense.

Inconsistent nutrition guidelines like this leave many people confused about what to eat after surgery. I have worked with many patients who report a chronic sense of guilt and a fear of weight-loss failure because they were just not able to follow radical recommendations like these. With a history of failed diet attempts people often end up feeling that it must be *them* doing something wrong. This is tragic! You have spent enough time agonizing over your weight. You don't need contradictory numbers that are impossible to follow; you need simple guidelines that work.

Comparing Your Owner's Manual Guidelines with the National Academy's of Science Institute of Medicine (IOM) Guidelines

Nutrient	Your Owner's Manual Guidelines	IOM Guidelines
Carbohydrate	30-33%	45-65%
Fat	33-34%	20-35%
Protein	34-36%	10-35%

By following your owner's manual guidelines, you can realistically balance food sources of carbohydrate, protein and fat while maximizing your weight loss. Restricting carbohydrate below this level would require increases in fat and protein to unhealthy and unrealistic proportions.

**300 – 400 Calorie Meals Comparing
Your Owner's Manual Guidelines with
Very Low Carbohydrate Diets (25g/day)**

For a range of 900-1,200 calories per day or 300-400 calories per meal, the breakdown would look like this:

300 Calorie Meal

Nutrient	Owner's Manual Guidelines % of Calories/grams	Fad Diet Guidelines % of Calories/grams
Carbohydrate	32% / 25g	11% / 8g
Fat *	33% / 11g	30% / 10g
Protein	35% / 26g (4oz.)	59% / 44g (6 oz.)

400 Calorie Meal

Nutrient	Owner's Manual Guidelines % of Calories/grams	Fad Diet Guidelines % of Calories/grams
Carbohydrate	32% / 32g	8% / 8g
Fat *	33% / 15g	23% / 10g
Protein	35% / 35g (5 oz.)	69% / 69g (10 oz.)

* **Note:** calories from fat were consistent for both groups using an appropriate budget of 10-15 grams per meal. Even if you increased the 400 calorie fad diet meal to 15 grams of fat, you would still have to eat 8 oz. of meat to consume enough calories (if total carbohydrate intake was restricted to 25 grams per day.)

A Snacking Exception

Some people report feeling very satisfied after eating moderate 300-400 calorie meals and report feelings of discomfort when eating portions larger than this. However, if the person's physical activity level and/or individual metabolism is/are high, eating just 900-1,200 calories per day may not be sufficient to meet their nutrition and energy needs. People in this situation may notice signs of fatigue, moodiness, lack of focus and cravings for sweets or other carbohydrates. These negative symptoms can be avoided while supporting appropriate weight loss for maintenance of current body weight by adding 1-3 protein-rich snacks (about 100-200 calories each) to the daily meal plan. See Table 26.2 and Appendix G for examples of appropriate protein-rich snacks.

Bottom Line: always follow the guidelines your surgeon, dietitian and medical-care team give you. Use the information provided in this chapter as a guideline while experimenting with what works best for you.

Table 26.2
Examples of Protein-Rich Snacks

Food	Portion Size	Protein	Calories
Boiled Egg	1 Large	7	75
Deli Meat	3 slices(1 oz. each)	21	75
Peanut Butter	1 Tablespoon	4	80
Almonds	1 oz. (12 nuts)	5	166
Cheddar Cheese	1 oz. Slice	7	114
Cottage Cheese	½ Cup	14	82

Note: to save calories, choose skim or 1% milk fat.

Twenty-seven

WHAT ABOUT HUNGER?

In This Chapter
- ◆ Understand that your appetite will increase gradually during the first few months up to about 2 years following surgery.
- ◆ Recognize reasons for eating other than physical hunger.
- ◆ Identify strategies for controlling emotional eating.
- ◆ Plan to maximize your window of opportunity and learn to out-smart weight loss plateaus.

Lack of Appetite

Most patients report the lowest appetite during the first six months to a year following surgery. Initially, it is common to hold only an ounce or two of food at a time because your stomach pouch will be swollen from surgery. You will be full and satisfied after eating very little food. This is often referred to as the "honeymoon phase" because most patients experience little hunger and the most rapid weight loss during this time. Choosing nutrient dense foods is essential to maximize weight loss and prevent nutrition related complications such as nausea, hair loss, or poor wound healing and frequent dumping.

Return of Appetite

After the initial swelling following surgery has subsided, it is normal to notice a gradual increase in appetite. Do not be alarmed – you have not "stretched" your pouch! However, it is important to know that you have a lot of control over how satisfied you feel following a meal, and how quickly your hunger will return again. Making appropriate food choices as part of your new lifestyle will determine whether or not you reach your goal weight and maintain the weight you have lost for a lifetime. Keep practicing the guidelines outlined in chapters 24 and 25; these truly are your keys to success.

Emotional Eating

Eating for reasons other than physical hunger is emotional eating. People unconsciously turn to food for comfort when bored, lonely, angry, sad, or in pain. Food is a friend. However, food used this way is like a drug; it is addictive.

Emotional eating is not a diet problem, but rather a *symptom* of other troubling issues that often leave people anxious or depressed. For example, it is common for people who have been victims of physical, sexual or emotional abuse to turn to food as a form of protection. Excess body weight may decrease the amount of attention received by others, thus leaving the person feeling safe.

Many people who eat for emotional reasons are not even aware of it. Yet it is essential to identify this behavior pattern so that it does not sabotage future weight loss efforts. If you eat for reasons other than hunger, consider seeking the support of a counselor who can assist you in working through the issues. Creating a healthy relationship with food is an essential part of any long-term weight-loss plan. (See Table 27.1 for strategies on managing emotional eating.)

Head Hunger

Head hunger refers to a perception of hunger sometimes reported by patients during the early post-op diet stages. These early sensations of hunger are not *physical hunger*. From past experience you associate a feeling of fullness in your belly with larger portions of food. Your new stomach pouch can only hold a small amount of food and the swelling following surgery limits this capacity even more. It is important to follow your surgeon's dietary guidelines during each stage of the post-op diet to avoid over-eating. Give your body time to learn new sensations of hunger and fullness. Feelings of head hunger typically pass soon after surgery.

Table 27.1
Strategies for Managing Emotional Eating

◆ **Remove yourself from the stressor.** Take ten deep breaths first. Whether you use breath work, or physically remove yourself from the environment, try to give yourself a fresh perspective on the source of your stress.

◆ **Plan ahead.** Write down at least five activities you could do instead of eating when you find yourself turning to food for comfort. Here are a few ideas to get you started: walk the dog; write in your journal; phone a friend; exercise; pick up a hobby like scrapbooking

◆ **Focus on all of your positive success.** This may help keep you strong and on the right path.

◆ **Snack on a protein-rich food if you do turn to food.** Since protein will fill you up quickly, you are less likely to eat too many calories or experience dumping.

Window of Opportunity

The first 6 to 12 months following surgery you will experience the most rapid weight loss and your greatest percentage of weight loss overall. You may hear this period of time referred to as your "window of opportunity." It is very important to maximize your weight loss during this time by eating adequate protein, making appropriate food choices and exercising regularly. These lifestyle changes will help you reach your goal weight and maintain your weight loss for a lifetime. I have observed time and again that the patients most likely to reach their goal weight are the ones who take advantage of this window of opportunity. Weight loss will never be this easy again.

Quick Tip: Make an emotional first aid kit. It's a list of things you can do that you know will make you feel better. That's what you should turn to when you're feeling emotional hunger.

Weight Loss Plateaus

Weight loss plateaus are periods of time when your weight loss slows down or stops temporarily. Early weight loss plateaus are often the result of your body trying to protect itself. Immediately following surgery your calorie intake is significantly lower than what your body was accustomed to. You start on a very low calorie liquid diet and progress to very small portions of semi-soft, then regular food over a period of 2-3 months. Most patients report a very low level of hunger during this time, often forgetting to eat. The body goes into a "starvation mode" when it senses this significant decrease in calories. This means your metabolism slows down and you may stop losing weight for a period of time.

Weight-loss plateaus can also occur later in your weight-loss journey, as you get closer to your goal weight. It takes less energy to do everyday activities when you weigh less. Your calorie requirement also is lower because you are burning fewer calories. Imagine putting weights into a backpack equal to the amount of body weight you have lost and carrying that around with you during the day. You would see very quickly that carrying extra body weight around requires a lot of energy!

Although weight loss plateaus are a normal bodily response, many patients report feeling discouraged when their weight loss slows or stops before reaching their goal weight. A common fear during weight-loss plateaus is that weight loss surgery will be just one more diet failure. This is simply not true.

Quick Tip: When you find yourself being self-critical, think about what you'd say to a friend if she was saying that about herself. You'd tell her it's no big deal, or that you love her anyway. Or you're confident she'll manage it and find the best solution. All right then, say those encouraging things to yourself.

The best approach to getting off a weight-loss plateau is to eat adequate protein and calories (do not under-eat) and maximize your lean body mass (muscle) through aerobic and resistance exercise. When the body is in "starvation mode" after eating too few calories it begins to break down muscle for energy. This breakdown has a slowing effect on the metabolism because it takes more calories to maintain muscle than it does to maintain fat. You want to preserve muscle at all costs. By consuming adequate protein and calories daily your body will not need to meet its nutrition needs by tearing down your muscles. This approach to dieting is often referred to as a protein sparing fast, meaning when you eat adequate protein and calories, muscle mass can be preserved because the body will not sense the threat of starvation. Be sure to eat adequate protein and calories, avoid skipping meals and regularly participate in both weight lifting and cardiovascular exercise to keep moving toward your goal weight. (See Chapter 31 for more on aerobic exercise and resistance training.)

Post-Chapter Exercises:

- *Exercise One:* If you are experiencing a weight-loss plateau, try something new. Your body gets used to the same old routine. When you mix things up a little bit, the new stimulation typically prompts your body into losing weight again. For example, if you always walk at the same speed and incline, try adding hills or alternate between walking and jogging. If you always walk on the treadmill, try the stationary bike, step-mill or elliptical trainer. See Chapter 31 for more ideas.
- *Exercise Two:* If you feel tempted to stress eat get moving instead. Exercise is a great stress reliever and antidepressant. Physical activity does not have to be formal exercise. Try jumping on a trampoline, in-line skating or playing in the yard with the kids.

Twenty-eight

NUTRITION SUPPORT AFTER BARIATRIC SURGERY

In This Chapter
+ Recognize that the type of bariatric procedure you have and your individual lab work determine the amount of nutrition support you need.
+ Identify the most common nutritional deficiencies after roux-en-Y gastric bypass surgery.
+ Understand the guidelines for nutrition supplementation.
+ Identify good food sources of the key nutrients discussed.

Determining Your Surgery Type

Bariatric surgery results in weight loss because it reduces the amount of calories you can consume and/or absorb. Surgical weight-loss procedures generally fall into three categories: restrictive procedures, malabsorptive procedures, or a combination of restrictive and malabsorptive procedures. Post-op nutrition support is specific to the type of weight loss surgery you have.

A **restrictive procedure**, such as the lap-band or vertical banded gastroplasty, simply reduces the amount of food you can hold in your stomach. Weight loss occurs because of smaller portion sizes and a decrease in total calorie intake. Nutrient deficiencies are less common with restrictive procedures. A daily multi-vitamin/mineral (MVI) supplement is recommended because you will be eating less food and getting fewer nutrients overall. Additional supplements are not standard, but are added based on individual need.

Complete digestion and absorption of the food we eat takes place in the small intestine (duodenum, jejunum and ileum). A **malabsorptive procedure** bypasses a portion of the small intestine (the duodenum and first portion of the jejunum). Thus fewer calories and nutrients are absorbed because food travels through a shorter span of your digestive tract.

A **combination procedure** both reduces the stomach size and bypasses a portion of the small intestine. You will feel full on smaller amounts of food *and* fewer of the calories and nutrients you eat are absorbed. The roux-en-y gastric bypass is a combination procedure and is currently the most common bariatric surgery performed.

> *Following weight loss surgery you will need to commit to a lifelong regimen of vitamin and mineral supplements daily.*

Nutrition Support

Regardless of which surgical procedure you had, you will be eating and/or absorbing less food and fewer nutrients. You will need to adjust your eating habits and commit to a daily regimen of vitamin and mineral supplements for the rest of your life following weight loss surgery. It is best to take a preventive approach with nutrition support because deficiencies occur over time and may result in irreversible damage by the time signs and symptoms present themselves. Many surgeons and bariatric programs recommend measuring patient's blood work every 3 to 4 months the first year following surgery and annually thereafter to ensure good nutrition status. The good news is you can expect good health if you monitor your blood work regularly and take your supplements daily. Always follow the nutrition guidelines given by your surgeon and registered dietitian.

Nutrition Support Following a Combination Procedure
Multi-Vitamin and Mineral Supplement (MVI)

A multi-vitamin and mineral supplement is recommended daily following surgery because you are eating less food and absorbing fewer nutrients from the foods you are eating. The Recommended Dietary Allowances (RDAs) indicate the minimum amount of vitamins and minerals advised for apparently healthy people. Be sure to take a supplement with a minimum of 100% of the essential vitamins and most minerals. The dose of a children's chewable vitamin may be increased to meet the nutritional requirements of an adult. Prenatal or high potency vitamins generally contain higher doses of iron and folate; these may be appropriate for use after surgery if you are anemic, pregnant, or trying to conceive. To avoid problems, complete follow-up lab work as recommended and discuss with your surgeon and/or dietitian to ensure your supplement regimen is appropriate for your individual needs.

> *Always follow your surgeon's guidelines for taking nutrition supplements and completing lab work follow up.*

For Best Absorption

The stoma, the opening between the pouch and the small intestine, is initially very narrow after surgery. This makes it difficult for particles larger than pea-sized to pass. Thus a large particle of food or a whole vitamin pill could potentially get lodged in this opening and cause some discomfort. Most patients start with a chewable MVI to avoid the uncomfortable situation of something "getting stuck."

Some surgeons allow patients to progress to a whole tablet about a year after surgery as the stoma gradually increases in diameter. This makes it more convenient for taking things like ibuprofen or acetaminophen for a headache. However, when taking your MVI, you may want to reconsider. It is more likely for an MVI in pill form to be poorly absorbed following surgery due to decreased exposure to gastric juices and less time for digestion and absorption due to bypassing a portion of the small intestine. For these reasons, I recommend patients stay with a chewable or liquid form of MVI for life to improve nutrient absorption.

Common Recommendations for Taking a Multivitamin-Mineral (MVI)

♦ Begin taking a MVI prior to surgery.
♦ Start a chewable or liquid MVI soon after surgery, as directed by your surgeon.
♦ Avoid time-release supplements.
♦ Take the chewable or liquid MVI with a meal to:
  a) reduce the risk of nausea and
  b) increase the absorption of fat soluble vitamins when eaten in the presence of a fat source.
♦ Continue a chewable or liquid MVI for life (do not switch to a whole tablet) to maximize absorption.

Iron

Iron deficiency anemia is common among weight-loss surgery patients. This is due in part to a poor diet prior to surgery, decreased intake of iron-rich foods during the initial post-op stages, and reduced iron absorption following surgery. Symptoms of iron deficiency anemia may include a drop in blood pressure, light-headedness, dizziness, weakness and an elevated pulse rate. More commonly, you will just feel very tired. It is not standard to take an iron supplement in addition to your daily MVI unless your bloodwork shows that you are anemic or you have a significant history of anemia. Always discuss your current lab values and any deficiency symptoms with your physician or dietitian before adding supplemental iron.

The best dietary sources of iron are clams, oysters and all meats. These foods are rich in heme iron, which is readily absorbed by the body. Vegetarian foods such as dark green, leafy vegetables, dried fruits, whole grain breads and cereals, legumes, nuts, seeds, soybeans and tofu contain non-heme iron, a form of iron that is not well absorbed. Foods rich in vitamin C food will aid the absorption of non-heme iron. Try topping your leafy green salad with slices of Vitamin C-rich tomatoes or oranges to increase iron absorption.

> **Some Factors Contributing to Iron Deficiency Anemia Following Surgery**
> * Poor diet quality and nutrition status prior to surgery.
> * Many iron-rich foods, like meat, nuts and seeds are very limited in the early stages of post-op diet, which reduces iron intake.
> * An acidic environment enhances iron absorption and gastric acid is reduced in the remaining stomach pouch.
> * The primary site of iron absorption is the duodenum, the first section of the small intestine, which is completely bypassed after surgery.

Vitamin B-12

Vitamin B-12 is necessary for optimal metabolism, proper nerve function and the production of red blood cells. Normally, gastric acid helps free B-12 from a supplement or food source. Intrinsic factor, a substance produced in the lining of the stomach, will then bind with B-12 in the duodenum, which allows the vitamin to later be absorbed in the distal ileum of the small intestine. B-12 is not well absorbed after weight loss surgery because of reduced production of gastric acid and limited contact with intrinsic factor. Vitamin B-12 should be a standard daily supplement after surgery with a 500 mcg sublingual (under the tongue) tablet or a monthly injection.

> *Gastric bypass patients have an increased risk for both iron and vitamin B12 deficiencies. At minimum, these lab values should be monitored pre-operatively and then annually, post-op.*

Folate

Many foods are rich in folate, including fruit, dried beans, orange juice, beef liver, dark green vegetables and whole grain breads and cereals. However, these foods are very limited in the early stages of the post-op diet. Poor dietary intake of folic acid, the potential for vitamin malabsorption, and any increase in stress all contribute to your need for supplemental folate following surgery.

Tips to Enhance the Absorption of Supplemental Iron
- Do *not* eat or drink calcium-rich products such as milk, yogurt, cheese or calcium-fortified orange juice with your iron supplement because calcium competes with iron for absorption.
- Supplemental calcium and calcium-rich foods should be consumed at least 3 hours apart from your iron supplement.
- Do not drink coffee and tea with your iron supplement; they decrease the absorption of iron.

Current research does not reflect folate malabsorption as a chronic nutritional concern. A standard MVI supplement contains 400 mcg of folate, which is adequate to correct low levels and prevent folate deficiency in most people. The Institute of Medicine panel recommends 800 mcg of folic acid as a safe upper limit. Supplemental doses greater than 1 mg of folic acid are discouraged because a high level of folate may mask a vitamin B-12 deficiency. Prenatal vitamins generally contain 1 mg of folate are not advised unless recommended by your physician or surgeon. The known role of folate in preventing neural tube defects makes consistent supplementation and monitoring in fertile women an important consideration. To avoid a folate deficiency, regularly eat foods rich in folic acid and take your MVI daily.

Calcium

Calcium is essential for many functions in the body including forming and preserving the health of bones and teeth, blood clotting, muscle contraction, regulating heart rate and releasing neurotransmitters (e.g. serotonin, norepinephrine and acetylcholine, which are chemicals in the brain). Calcium supplements taken during any type of weight loss are critical for optimizing calcium absorption and the body's tissue reserves.

After bariatric surgery, calcium is an especially important nutrient to supplement. Calcium is preferentially absorbed in the duodenum and upper jejunum of the small intestine where the environment is more acidic. Also, calcium absorption is dependent on Vitamin D to activate a calcium-binding protein in the small intestine. Thus an alkaline (non-acidic) environment and malabsorption of Vitamin D following surgery both decrease the amount of calcium that is absorbed.

Another important consideration for calcium and bone health is the natural decline in estrogen in both men and women as we age. Lower estrogen levels result in less calcium absorbed by the intestine and kidneys. This signals bone to slow construction and speed up demolition. As women go through menopause, unless they take supplemental estrogen, most lose bone at a rapid rate of about 1 - 3 percent per year. About four to eight years after the onset of menopause, bone loss slows to an average of 1 percent per year. Declining estrogen levels does weaken bone in men as they age, although it is at a lower rate of about 1 percent per year.

> *"Optimum levels of calcium, vitamin D and physical activity are important for bone health."*
> *— The Surgeon General*

Some other reasons to supplement with calcium include possible lactose intolerance leading to poor dietary intake, or simply not including calcium-rich foods in the diet regularly. High sodium or caffeine intake and heavy sweating from exercise or work increases calcium excretion. Supplements with large amounts of any single mineral, such as magnesium, zinc, phosphorous, silicon, boron and iron, interfere with calcium absorption unless all the minerals are in balance. Finally, health conditions such as Crohn's and celiac disease, liver disorders and steatorrhea (fat malabsorption) increase your need for calcium.

> *"A negative balance of only 50-100 mg of calcium per day over a long period of time is sufficient to produce osteoporosis."*
> *— The Surgeon General*

When you are not taking in enough calcium from food (or a supplement) your body will pull calcium from your bones and teeth, because this is where 99 percent of the body's calcium is stored. Effects of a calcium deficiency may include muscle cramping, irregular heart rate, impaired blood clotting, weight gain, hypertension, and increased risk of bone fracture. The recommended daily intake of calcium is 1,000 mg for people age 19-50 and 1,200 – 1,500 mg for persons over 50 years of age. A negative balance of only 50-100 mg of calcium per day over a long period of time is sufficient to produce osteoporosis.

Calcium-Rich Foods

Food	*Amount of Calcium*
Milk, 1 Cup	300 mg
Tofu, ½ Cup, raw, firm	258 mg
Cheddar Cheese, 1 oz.	204 mg
Salmon, 3 oz. (canned w/bone)	203 mg
Yogurt, 6 oz.	200 mg
Mozzarella Cheese, 1 oz.	163 mg
Cottage Cheese, 1 Cup	138 mg
Broccoli, 1 Cup (cooked)	94 mg
Almonds, 1 oz.	80 mg
Oysters, 6 Medium	68 mg
Almond Butter, 1 Tbsp.	43 mg
Clams, 4 Large or 9 Small	40 mg

Considerations for Supplementing Calcium

+ Calcium citrate is often recommended over calcium carbonate because calcium citrate does *not* require an acidic environment in order to be absorbed. Although still a topic of clinical debate, several studies have shown calcium citrate is better absorbed by 22 percent to 27 percent, compared to calcium carbonate, whether it was taken on an empty stomach or with meals. Taking calcium citrate over other forms of supplemental calcium may prove to have greater health benefits without any known risks.

+ Take 1,000-1,500 mg Calcium Citrate with Vitamin D daily in a chewable or liquid form.

- Space calcium supplements and calcium-rich foods throughout the day. Doses up to 500 mg appear to be better absorbed than higher doses.
- Do not combine calcium supplements or calcium rich foods with supplements containing iron because they compete for absorption.
- Monitor your blood work closely if you currently take, or have a history of taking, anti-seizure or glucocorticoid medications, as these medications may increase your need for calcium.

Supplements at a Glance

Nutrient	*Recommended For*	*Amount*
Iron	*Menstruating Females and those at high risk (e.g. adolescents, anemia or if anemia develops after surgery)*	325 mg ferrous sulfate (65 mg elemental iron) in addition to daily MVI *pre-op*
Folate	*All Post-Op Patients*	A daily MVI containing 400-800 mcg
	Fertile women and persons with a known folate deficiency	A Prenatal or high potency MVI with 1,000 mcg of folate daily
Vitamin B12	*All Post-Op Patients*	500 mcg/day OR 1,000 mcg injection/mo.
Calcium	*All Post-Op Patients*	1,000-1,500 mg calcium with Vitamin D (in several doses no > 500 mg/ each)
Vitamin D	*All Post-Op Patients*	A daily MVI with 400 IU (10 mcg)

Vitamin B1 (Thiamine)

While some vitamin malabsorption is expected after bariatric surgery, a low thiamine level should *not* be a common concern. Frequent vomiting can lead to an acute thiamine deficiency. So be sure to monitor your blood work following any vomiting episode. Severe restriction of foods high in B-vitamins and/or poor compliance with daily MVI supplement may result in a late thiamine deficiency (known as beriberi). Early signs of deficiency include fatigue, irritability, sensitivity to noise, memory loss, inability to concentrate, sleep disturbances, appetite loss, slow wound healing, depression and constipation. To avoid a vitamin B1 deficiency take your MVI daily and regularly eat foods rich in thiamine and other B vitamins, such as lean pork, beef, liver, brewer's yeast, peas, beans, brown rice and whole or enriched grains and bread. Thiamine levels should be assessed preoperatively and then annually in the non-complicated patient.

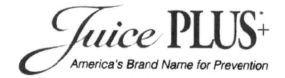

America's Brand Name for Prevention

The Only Exception to the "No Juice Rule" After Gastric Bypass Surgery

When you cut an apple slice and leave it on the counter, it turns brown. This is a visible sign of oxidation. In a similar way the cells in your body continually endure oxidative stress from the activity of free radicals.

Free radicals are highly reactive molecules created within your body when it burns fuel for energy or with exposure to cigarette smoke, environmental pollutants, asbestos, radiation, excessive alcohol consumption, poor diet and bacterial, fungal or viral infections. Oxidative damage has been implicated in the cause of certain diseases and has an impact on the body's aging process.

It's the job of antioxidants to neutralize free radicals. By eating a diet rich in antioxidants you can help your body defend itself against oxidative stress.

Fruits and vegetables contain a variety of powerful antioxidants. The current USDA recommendations are to include 9-13 servings of fruit and vegetables in the diet daily (see: www.mypyramid.gov). Many people were not meeting the previous, lower guidelines of 5 servings per day and if you've had gastric bypass surgery the challenge to meet this daily goal is even greater.

> The best source of antioxidants is *not* an isolated vitamin or a specific antioxidant. The best source is whole food!

Juice Plus+® provides whole food based nutrition from 17 different fruits, vegetables and grains – plus fiber blends – in convenient capsule, chewable or gummie forms. Juice Plus+® is the only nutrition supplement I take daily and I insist that my husband, parents and siblings take it, too. I feel comfortable recommending Juice Plus+® to my patients because there is a large and growing body of independent, peer reviewed research which shows:

- Juice Plus+® is packed with concentrated whole food nutrition.
- Juice Plus+® raises levels of antioxidants in the blood.
- Juice Plus+® lowers levels of lipid peroxides and homocysteine in the blood.
- Juice Plus+® helps enhance immune function, reduce DNA damage and improve circulation.

For more information or to order Juice Plus+®, visit www.KatNutrition.com.

Post-Chapter Exercises:

- *Exercise One:* If you have trouble remembering to take your vitamin supplements regularly, try putting them in a place that could help remind you such as by your toothbrush, next to the coffee pot or by your car keys.
- *Exercise Two:* Choose three calcium-rich foods you like and include them with your meals this week.
- *Exercise Three:* Monitor your records and plan ahead to schedule your next lab work check-up.

Twenty-Nine

SPECIAL CONSIDERATIONS

In This Chapter
- Understand lactose intolerance and appropriate dietary changes to ease symptoms.
- Differentiate between behavioral and anatomical reasons for vomiting.
- Identify strategies for minimizing nausea, vomiting, constipation, diarrhea, food blockages, muscle cramps, hair loss and depression.
- Understand that meat is an important protein source and a variety of meats should be included in your post-op diet.
- Learn tips to increase your ability to tolerate a variety of meats.
- Learn strategies for eating out after surgery.

Nausea and Vomiting

Mild nausea is relatively common the first few months following surgery as you adjust to your new pouch and progress through the initial diet stages. Follow your surgeon's guidelines and try some of the suggestions in Table 29.1 to reduce the frequency and ease symptoms of nausea.

Vomiting, on the other hand, should *not* be a common problem after surgery. There are several things to consider while determining the cause of chronic vomiting. Some of these causes include: a stricture or blockage, an ulcer, gallstones, gastritis, sinus drainage, pregnancy and food poisoning. Dehydration, acute thiamine deficiency and other complications from chronic vomiting can be serious, so call your surgeon right away if vomiting is persistent. Common, less serious causes for vomiting are typically behavioral reasons that can be modified (See Table 29.2)

Table 29.1
Minimizing Nausea
- Follow your surgeon's guidelines for adding foods back to the diet one stage at a time.
- Eat slowly and chew food thoroughly.
- Moist foods are typically tolerated better than dry foods.
- Avoid fatty foods, or too much fat at one meal.
- Keep a food diary to track problem foods.
- Try sipping ginger, chamomile or peppermint tea.

Table 29.2
Vomiting: Behavioral Reasons
- Eating too fast
- Not chewing food thoroughly before swallowing
- Eating too much
- Adding a food back to the diet too early
- Drinking fluids with meals
- Eating very dry foods
- Reclining too soon after a meal (less than one hour)

Lactose Intolerance

Lactose is a sugar molecule found naturally in milk and dairy products composed of the two simple sugars glucose and galactose. People who are lactose intolerant lack or have a low level of the enzyme lactase which breaks down lactose during digestion. The inability to digest lactose can result in bloating, gas, cramping and diarrhea when eating dairy products. Even if you have never had a problem with milk products before, you may experience lactose intolerance after bariatric surgery because the lactase enzyme is found in the duodenum, the bypassed portion of the small intestine. People with no prior history of lactose intolerance may find that their symptoms will improve or disappear several months to a few years after surgery as the gut adapts to its new anatomy.

Tips for Dealing with Lactose Intolerance

- Try reduced lactose products such as "Lactaid" brand dairy products that are treated with the lactase enzyme.
- Try a non-dairy substitute like soy yogurt, soy cheese and soy based protein powders that don't contain lactose.
- Chew an over-the-counter lactase enzyme tablet with the first bite of dairy food.
- People with mild lactose intolerance often do well with regular dairy yogurt and hard cheeses, which have lower levels of lactose.
- The symptoms of lactose intolerance can mimic those of dumping. Be sure to consider the grams of carbohydrate from dairy products when determining your total carbohydrates per meal.

Muscle Cramps

Some common causes of muscle cramping are poor fluid intake, acute dehydration from diarrhea, vomiting or excessive sweating, medications that increase urinary excretion of potassium and/or low dietary intake of potassium. Be sure to drink adequate fluids, take your MVI daily, and increase your intake of potassium by including dark green vegetables, tropical fruits and salt substitutes in your diet on a regular basis. (See Spinach Salad Recipe in Appendix H.) Consult your surgeon or registered dietitian before supplementing with potassium.

Bad Breath

If you have attempted weight loss in the past on a low carbohydrate diet, you may remember experiencing a chronic, metallic taste similar to a cross between nail polish remover and over-ripe pineapple. This occurs in dieters who put themselves in a state of ketosis by consuming very little carbohydrate. Ketosis occurs when your blood sugar drops so low that your body has to break down stored fat to make glucose. Bad breath is a temporary side effect of weight loss surgery. As you progress into your maintenance diet and are able to eat more carbohydrates and more calories in general, ketosis and bad breath should subside.

Changes in Taste

Many patients report that food just doesn't taste the same after surgery. This is more commonly reported with taste sensitivity to sweets, which often taste "too sweet" following surgery. This can be an advantage for patients who had cravings for sweets and other junk foods prior to surgery. Research supports patient reported taste variations following gastric bypass surgery, but the cause of these changes is not known. Remember to keep an open mind when adding new foods to your diet. Alterations in your taste buds may make it easier for you to give up some of your old food habits and begin healthier ones.

Constipation

The initial post-op diet poses the greatest challenge with constipation because it is low in fiber, low in calories, high in protein and often too low in fluids. See Table 29.3 for tips on minimizing constipation.

Diarrhea

You may experience moderate diarrhea initially after surgery due to the changes in your diet and digestive track. Follow the guidelines for minimizing constipation and avoid foods that are high in fat, sugar, lactose and caffeine to improve symptoms. Be conscious of possible dehydration and consult your surgeon if diarrhea becomes chronic.

Getting Food Stuck

For the first year following roux-en-y gastric bypass, the stoma or opening between the stomach pouch and the small intestine is very small. Vitamins and medications must be crushed or chewed the first year post-op, and food must be chewed thoroughly to avoid becoming lodged or stuck. Over time, the stoma expands. About a year after surgery, small tablets can be swallowed whole and there is less risk of food particles blocking the pouch opening. If food does become blocked in your stoma it will usually work its way through, or dissolve by itself. However, this process can be painful, and may take several hours to subside. Take your time when eating meals and chew your food thoroughly before swallowing. See Table 29.4 for tips on avoiding a food blockage.

Table 29.3
Tips for Alleviating Constipation
- Drink an adequate amount of water.
- Eat regular meals to optimize metabolism and keep your bowels moving.
- Choose high-fiber foods such as vegetables, fruit, beans and whole grains when eating carbohydrates.
- Aim for 20-35 grams of fiber per day.
- Encourage your body's natural elimination process by avoiding stimulant laxatives.
- Try an over the counter bulk-forming laxative (BeneFiber™, Metamucil™ or Citrucel™) that draws water into the colon and softens the stool.
- Exercise regularly.
- Consider taking a probiotic supplement (e.g. Lactobacillus Acidophilus, the culture found in yogurt) to optimize the healthy bacteria in your colon promoting regularity.

Table 29.4
Tips on Avoiding a Food Blockage:
- Eat slowly and chew your food thoroughly.
- During the early stages of your post-op diet avoid foods like rice and soft bread that tend to get "gummy" when mixed with saliva or very dry foods (like over-cooked meats) which are more likely to get lodged in the stoma.
- Be cautious when eating fibrous foods such as asparagus, celery, cooked spinach, broccoli, popcorn and the skins of apples or cucumbers.

Hair Loss

Many women report hair loss after giving birth, and some bariatric patients experience moderate hair loss in the early stages after surgery. Hair loss in these situations is considered to be a normal bodily response to stress and is typically short term (occurring within 3 months of surgery). However, hair loss that occurs later than 3 months post-op indicates protein mal-nutrition. This is a more serious nutritional deficiency and is often accompanied by leg edema (swelling of the lower legs) and deficiencies of other vitamins and minerals. The best approach for minimizing your chances of early or late hair loss is to start an MVI prior to surgery, regularly take all nutritional supplements recommended by your surgeon, and meet your goal for protein daily.

> *Some patients report easing the symptoms of a food blockage by chewing a digestive enzyme tablet, such as papaya ... or slowly sipping on warm water with a touch of meat tenderizer, for a blockage involving meat.*

Losing Too Much Weight

Although not as common as some of the other considerations discussed in this chapter, losing too much weight is a challenge for some post-op patients. If your goal is weight gain because you are losing below your goal weight, the best approach is to add 1 – 2 protein-rich snacks daily to increase your calorie intake. Using meal replacement drinks, eating small frequent meals and eating more carbohydrates and less protein at each meal will also result in weight *gain* because all three of these strategies will increase your calorie intake without making you feel too full. Choose the most conservative approach first, making additional changes as needed. Be careful to monitor your weight closely to prevent too much weight gain.

Table 29.5
Identifying More Serious Signs of Depression
- Feeling hopeless, irritable or restless
- Mood changes such as anger and frequent crying
- Inability to sleep or sleeping excessively
- Feelings of low self-worth
- Chronic feelings of sadness that don't go away
- A complete disinterest in things that used to interest you
- Thoughts of death or suicide

Depression

Depression is nothing to be ashamed of. There are many reasons for depression following surgery and many people struggled with the condition prior to surgery. It is relatively common to experience some unhappy feelings soon after surgery as your body recovers, and you adjust to your new lifestyle. Initially you will feel tired and lethargic, you may experience some pain as you recuperate or some nausea when drinking or eating. Don't focus on the short-term. This is a time to lean on your family and friends for support and keep your mind focused on positive things. Your surgery is behind you and you are starting to lose weight; you can breathe easier, move around better and are probably already coming off of some of your medications. Consider some of the tips in Table 29.6 for "Saying Good-bye to the Blues." If you identify with any of the characteristics in table 29.5, "Identifying More Serious Signs of Depression," discuss your symptoms with your physician and consider seeking additional support from a counselor to ensure your health and weight loss success.

If you're feeling down, talk to someone. Your family, friends, surgeon, nurse, dietitian, counselor and support group are good places to start.

Table 29.6
Saying "Good-bye" to the Blues

+ *Focus on the positive*; you are starting a whole new phase of your life!
+ *Adjust your mind-set*; set realistic goals and expectations.
+ *Surround yourself with positive friends and family.*
+ *Get Moving!* exercise is one of the best natural anti-depressants. As soon as your doctor gives you the O.K., start with a low impact aerobic activity like walking, swimming, cycling or the elliptical trainer and progress from there.
+ *Get adequate Zzzzzzs.* getting eight hours of sleep each night will positively affect your mood and ability to concentrate.
+ *Give yourself good nutrition support* – follow your surgeon's dietary guidelines, take your vitamin supplements daily and drink adequate fluids.
+ *Listen to music that lifts your spirits.*
+ *Attend support group regularly.*
+ *Try aromatherapy* scents that make you smile inside
+ *Fill your prescription for 15 minutes of laughter daily.*
+ *Nurture your spiritual side.*

For more information on depression call your surgeon and visit the National Institute of Mental Health's web-site at *www.nimh.nih.gov/publicat/depression.cfm#ptdep3.*

Eating Out

Eating out can be a very appropriate part of your post-op lifestyle. Below are some tips for dining out as part of your maintenance diet.

Tips for Dining Out Bariatric Style

+ *Consider an appetizer for your entrée.* Many appetizers are high in protein, appropriately portioned and easy to eat. Ideas: shrimp cocktail, lobster tails or crab cakes.

- *When in doubt, order eggs.* They are a great source of protein and are sure to fill you up.
- *Don't order off the children's menu just because the portions are smaller.* Pizza, chicken nuggets and macaroni & cheese are not the best food choices. It would be better to order a protein-rich entrée in a larger portion and take the leftovers home. So enjoy yourself and choose something you like.
- *Limit temptation and unwanted questions.* Plan ahead and ask the wait staff for a "to go" bag when placing your order. This will decrease your chances of over-eating and may prevent un-wanted questions about your diet or if there was something wrong with your food.
- *At specialty restaurants stick with protein-rich choices* such as Italian meatballs, Mexican fajitas and Chinese chicken and vegetables without rice.
- *Always ask that sauces be served "on the side"* and consider the sugar, fat and calories in sauces and dressings.
- *Choose the tenderest cuts of meat* such as fillet mignon and pork tenderloin. You may even want to request a specific cooking temperature for your meat entrees (see Table 29.7.)
- *When uncertain about a new food choice,* don't over-do it. Try a small portion and see how well you tolerate it before eating more.

Eating Meat

When adding meat back to the post-op diet many programs start with the addition of fish first because it is light, flaky and easy to chew and swallow. Chicken is typically added back to the diet a week later followed by pork and red meat. Most programs encourage patients to eat foods from all food groups by 2-3 months following surgery, includ-ing a variety of meats. However, patients commonly associate meat with negative symptoms such as getting food stuck or vomiting. Don't stop reading here, there's more to the story!

Food preparation is a very important consideration when eating meat after surgery. Cooking methods that enhance the moisture content of a meat will increase your ability to tolerate it well. When preparing meat be sure to use a food thermometer and consult the temperature guide-lines provided in Table 29.7. Using appropriate cooking temperatures specific to the type of meat you are preparing protects you against food borne illness from under-cooked meats and decreases the likelihood of over-cooking and drying-out your entrée. The result? A moist, enjoyable piece of meat. You may also want to consider the following:

- *Choose tender cuts of meat* such as top loin, tenderloin, sirloin or T-bone steak and the dark meat of chicken and turkey.
- *Choose the least expensive, chuck ground beef* because it's higher fat content makes the meat more moist.
- *Match the cooking method to the cut of meat.* Dry heat cooking methods are appropriate only for very tender cuts of meat. Longer, moist methods of cooking are best for less tender cuts of meat to enhance the break-down of connective tissues. Marinating, pounding with a meat mallet and slicing across the grain are other techniques for treating tougher cuts of meat.
- *Use broth, sauces and gravies to add moisture* to meat. Keep an eye on fat and sugar content to avoid dumping symptoms and excessive calories.
- *Don't over-cook your meat.* Use a meat thermometer and the guidelines below for cooking meat to a safe temperature while maintaining optimum moisture.
- *Dust off your crock-pot.* Moist, slow-cook methods are an excellent way to keep meats moist and juicy.

Table 29.7
Minimum Safe Internal Cooking Temperatures for Preparing Moist Meats
Insert a meat thermometer into the center of the meat to measure its internal cooking temperature.

Food Product	*Minimum Safe Internal Cooking Temperatures in degrees Fahrenheit (F)*
Poultry	165° F
Beef	155° F
Pork	145° F
Fish	140° F

Post-Chapter Exercises:

- *Exercise One:* If you are experiencing symptoms of lactose intolerance try over-the-counter lactase enzyme tablets, milk treated with the lactase enzyme (e.g. Lactaid brand milk) or non-dairy soy products.

- *Exercise Two:* Take advantage of your taste bud changes and experiment with a new food this week, even if it is something you did not like in the past.

- *Exercise Three:* Buy a meat thermometer and experiment cooking your meats to optimize moisture content and taste. You will be amazed how much more you will enjoy meat!

- *Exercise Four:* When eating out this week, try choosing a protein-rich appetizer, like shrimp cocktail, as your entrée.

Thirty

FLUID FACTS

In This Chapter
- Understand the Institute of Medicine's guidelines for daily water intake.
- Identify foods and fluids that support hydration.
- Recognize signs of dehydration.
- Identify fluids to avoid.
- Know what to consider when drinking caffeine and alcohol.

Key Words to Know
- *Dehydration:* occurs when the concentration of solid particles in the blood rises by 5 percent due to inadequate fluid intake or losses such as excessive sweating, vomiting or diarrhea.

Liquid Assets

Most people are familiar with the old "8 x 8" rule of aiming to drink 64 oz. of water daily. What many people may not realize is that much more than plain water counts toward this goal. In February 2004 the National Academies' Institute of Medicine revised its recommendations for water intake. After reviewing more than 400 studies the authors set the general daily intake for women at approximately 91 ounces (2.7 Liters) and for men at about 125 ounces (3.7 Liters.) This may sound like a lot, but these numbers include fluids from both food and water.

About 80 percent of people's water intake comes from drinking water and other beverages, including caffeinated drinks; the other 20 percent is derived from food. Even pasta is 66 percent water (see Table 30.1)

Table 30.1
Water Content of Selected Foods

Food	% Water
Apple	86
Banana	75
Bread, whole wheat	38
Cheese, Cheddar	37
Cottage Cheese	79
Chicken, roasted	64
Crackers, Saltines	4
Grapes	81
Ham, cooked	70
Lettuce, iceberg	96
Pasta	66
Peanuts, dry roasted	2
Potato, baked	75
Steak, tenderloin	50
Turkey, roasted	62
Walnuts	4

Source: National Academy of Sciences, *Dietary Reference Intakes for Water, Potassium, Sodium, Chloride and Sulfate.* February 11, 2004.

Bottoms Up

Your daily water needs will not change following surgery, but the way you consume your fluids *will*. Because you will be eating less food in general, water from food will make a smaller contribution toward your daily goal. This increases the importance of drinking adequate fluids after surgery. You should plan to meet your fluid needs by sipping on liquids throughout the day in between meals. See Table 30.2 for tips on meeting your daily fluid goal.

The first few months following surgery can be a challenging time for getting enough fluids because post-operative swelling restricts what your new stomach pouch can hold. It is important that you plan ahead, sip on fluids throughout the day and do your best to stay hydrated.

Dehydration occurs when the concentration of solid particles in the blood rises by 5 percent, meaning there is less fluid to separate the particles. Thirst is triggered when blood concentrations rise by 2 percent. Thus, thirst is the first indicator of the body's need for water. Don't wait for thirst, though. Plan ahead and drink appropriate fluids throughout the day.

Poor hydration often results from acute episodes of vomiting. Although only a small number of people experience vomiting after surgery, dehydration can occur quickly and could require intravenous fluids. Always seek medical attention if vomiting is persistent.

The most common signs and symptoms of dehydration include persistent fatigue, headaches, muscle cramps, nausea, light-headedness, confusion, dry skin and increased heart rate. If you experience any of these symptoms, try to determine if the cause is poor fluid intake.

Another side effect of poor hydration is an increased appetite. In other words, if you feel hungry, it may be your body's way of signaling thirst. Remember food typically contributes about 20% of your daily need for fluid. After surgery you will be eating less, thus getting less fluid from your diet overall. It's common to crave certain foods or have a higher appetite in general when not drinking enough as the body tries to compensate for the fluid it needs. Obviously this is not ideal for people who are trying to lose or maintain their current body weight. Be sure to drink adequate fluids daily to optimize your metabolism and keep unwanted cravings at bay.

Considering Caffeine

A study published in the *Journal of the American College of Nutrition* debunked the myth that caffeinated beverages zap your body's water reserves. "I worked with elite-level athletes ... and noticed they drank a lot of caffeinated beverages without showing any sign of dehydration," says Ann Grandjean, Ph.D., a hydration researcher, consultant to the United States Olympic Committee and executive director of the non-profit Center for Human Nutrition in Omaha, Nebraska. Grandjean and colleagues recruited 18 healthy men for their hydration study. The men were given 59 fluid ounces of liquid including water, diet soda and coffee in varying amounts based on the subject's body mass. Each participant's body weight, urine and blood were tested before and after drinking the fluids. Researchers found that the body doesn't discriminate between regular and decaffeinated beverages when it comes to hydration. It appears that the diuretic effect of caffeine does not produce a greater fluid loss overall; however, the length of time between consuming and excreting fluid through the urine can be slightly shorter when drinking caffeinated beverages compared to caffeine-free fluids.

Table 30.2
Tips for Meeting Your Daily Fluid Goal
- **Plan ahead.** Carry a water bottle with you.
- **Take small sips of fluid** every few minutes in between meals to meet your daily fluid goal.
- **Remember all calorie-free, non-carbonated fluids contribute toward your fluid goal.** Try a variety of appropriate drinks to find several that you like.
- **Be consistent.** As your body gets used to proper hydration, you will be able to feel the difference when you are not drinking enough.
- **Avoid alcohol** to limit excess calories and improve overall hydration.

There are still good reasons to moderate or discontinue your caffeine intake after surgery. Here are a few things to consider:

- **Caffeine increases the amount of calcium excreted in your urine.** Maintaining a positive calcium balance is a common nutrition concern after bariatric surgery. That's why it is not advisable to increase your calcium needs further with excessive caffeine intake.
- **Caffeine can be irritating to the gastro-intestinal tract, including your new stomach pouch.** Avoid caffeine the first 6 months after surgery and consume in moderation if you decide to add it back later in your maintenance diet.

- **Consider your blood pressure and anxiety level.** Caffeine is a stimulant and can increase your heart rate, blood pressure and feelings of anxiety. If you are currently taking medications for anxiety or hypertension you may want to consider limiting or discontinuing caffeine to improve your overall symptoms.
- **Make note of your appetite.** Some people report increased or decreased appetite when consuming caffeine. This can interfere with your weight-loss goals when an increased appetite leads to eating extra calories or a decreased appetite results in skipping meals and slowing the metabolism. Decrease caffeine intake if it interferes with your normal appetite.
- **Get a good night's sleep.** Caffeine stays in your system for 12 hours. So if you are drinking caffeine for a 3:00 p.m. pick-me-up that caffeine will stay with you until 3:00 a.m. Even if you don't feel anxious or revved up, the residual effect of caffeine can keep you from reaching deeper levels of restful sleep, leaving you tired and lethargic in the morning.

The Bubbly Stuff

Carbonated drinks like diet soda, sparkling water and champagne will cause more gas and bloating after surgery because there is less room in the stomach for gas to dissipate. Even more alarming, recent studies demonstrate an increased rate of weight re-gain in patients who resume carbonated drinks when compared to similar patients who do not. Although current research supporting the relationship between carbonated drinks and weight re-gain is non-conclusive, it may be in your best interest to refrain from the bubbly stuff. In my practice I see a lot of variation among surgeons and bariatric programs on recommendations for consuming or avoiding carbonated drinks. Bottom line: always follow the guidelines given by your sugeon and stay advised of current evidence-based research specific to the post-gastric bypass lifestyle.

How About a Cocktail?

You'll be able to drink alcohol after surgery, but plan on less frequent and smaller portions. Because you have lower levels of the enzyme alcohol dehydrogenase, alcohol gets into your bloodstream much faster. One alcoholic drink typically has the effect of 2 or 3. This is also more toxic on your liver. Here are some things to keep in mind when drinking:

Table 30.3
Low Carbohydrate Cocktails:

You won't believe these cocktails are all less
than 4 grams of carbohydrate per serving!

Strawberry-Orange Daiquiri
(3 carbohydrates)
1 and ½ oz. rum
1 Tbsp. orange brandy
1 and ½ oz. lime juice
1 oz. sugar free orange syrup
2 large strawberries
4 ice cubes

Caribbean Cream
(2 carbohydrates)
2 oz. Caribbean Rum
2 oz. cream
1 tsp. Splenda
4 ice cubes

Walk the Red Carpet
(1.75 carbohydrates)
1 oz. tequila
1 and ½ oz. Caribbean Rum
4 oz. diet V8 Splash strawberry-kiwi
½ tsp. strawberry SF Kool-Aid
½ tsp. Splenda
4 ice cubes

Blueberry Buzz
(1.5 carbohydrates)
1 oz. whiskey
1 oz. chilled espresso
(or strong instant coffee)
4 oz. low carb, reduced
- fat chocolate milk
4 ice cubes

*To prepare any of the drink recipes above, combine all ingredients
in a blender and blend until smooth. Pour, drink and enjoy!*

- **Avoid alcohol at least 6 months to a year after surgery.** The empty calories may thwart your weight loss goals and cause other nutrition complications, such as dehydration, poor thiamine status and other forms of malnutrition when fluids, vitamins and minerals are replaced with alcohol.
- **Stay away from high carbohydrate drinks** like margaritas and daiquiris to avoid a rapid onset of dumping symptoms. (See Table 30.3 for a list of lower carbohydrate cocktails.)
- **Introduce alcohol in a safe environment.** Alcohol will affect you differently after surgery so imbibe with caution as you learn your new drinking limits.
- **Do not drink and drive.** Whether you have had the surgery or not you should always check your blood alcohol level before driving if you have been drinking. After surgery, however, you may be surprised to find how quickly your blood alcohol level will rise with just one small drink.
- **Separate your liquids and solids.** Treat alcohol like any other fluid: stop drinking 15-30 minutes before eating and wait an hour after a meal before resuming fluids.
- **Consider your liver.** If you have current or past medical history of any liver disorders, be very cautious with the use of alcohol after bariatric surgery.

Post-Chapter Exercises:

- *Exercise One:* Buy a pre-measured water bottle and carry it with you during the day to make fluid-tracking easier.
- *Exercise Two:* Consider decreasing or discontinuing caffeine if you struggle with a very low appetite during the day, causing you to under-eat or if you frequently have difficulty sleeping at night. Both of these behaviors will negatively impact your weight loss and weight loss maintenance.
- *Exercise Three:* At your next social event involving alcohol, try substituting a low carbohydrate cocktail (see Table 30.3) in place of your higher carbohydrate choices of the past.

Thirty-one

LEARNING TO ENJOY EXERCISE – NO SOAP BOX HERE

In This Chapter
- Identify the 5 basic components of fitness.
- Understand 3 variables for overcoming fitness plateaus.
- Recognize the importance of a good support system.
- Creative ideas to help you get started and stay motivated.

Key Words to Know
- **Muscular Strength:** the ability to exert maximum force, usually in a single repetition (e.g. one lift on the bench press with maximum weight.)
- **Muscular Endurance:** the ability to repeat an activity many times (e.g. one hundred abdominal crunches.)
- **Aerobic:** in the presence of oxygen; aerobic exercise involves continuous rhythmic movements over an extended period of time (e.g. walking or swimming.)
- **Anaerobic:** not in the presence of oxygen; anaerobic exercise involves short bursts of movement such as a sprint or lifting weights.
- **Strength or Resistance Training:** an anaerobic form of exercise that involves progressively lifting increasing amounts of weights to develop the strength and size of skeletal muscles.

(Continued on next page)

> ◆ **A Repetition:** completing both the lifting and lowering phase of an exercise one time; referred to as "a rep."
> ◆ **A Set:** a group of consecutive repetitions, typically followed by a brief rest period.
> ◆ **Body Composition:** the proportion of your body's make-up including body fat and lean body mass such as muscle, bone, skin and water.
> ◆ **Overload:** a principle that states a greater load or stress is required to continue making improvements in fitness once the body has adapted to the initial stress.

Reality Check

Let's face it – you don't need me to tell you that physical activity is good for you or that you *should* be exercising. Yet a surprising 66% of Americans do not exercise. Time is the number one excuse people report for not working out. In this chapter we will discuss the 5 basic components of fitness: muscular strength, muscular endurance, cardiovascular fitness, flexibility and body composition. We will then address a few personal topics, such as strategies for overcoming exercise barriers, setting short and long-term goals, designing your own exercise program, the importance of a good support system and tips to increase your motivation.

> **Examples of Physical Activities with Varying Intensity**
>
> | *Mild* | *Moderate* | *Vigorous* |
> |---|---|---|
> | Walking the dog | Cycling | Jogging (10min./mi.) |
> | Watering the plants | Gardening | Jumping Rope |
> | Ballroom dancing | Golf (no cart) | Tennis |

How Much is Enough?

The Institute of Medicine (IOM) recommends that adults and children alike should engage in activities equivalent to a total of 60 minutes of moderately intense physical activity daily. Compared to the more conservative goal set by the Surgeon General's report in 1996, to exercise a minimum of 20-30 minutes, 3 days per week, the IOM's recommendations for physical activity may seem a little daunting. But keep in mind this 60-minute goal includes all physical activity throughout the day, not just formal exercise. So gardening, walking the dog and light housekeeping are all activities that contribute toward a fit lifestyle. Get more active today with short-term goals such as parking further away from your destination and walking (for more ideas, see Table 31.1)

Table 31.1
Simple Steps to Becoming More Active

Get off the bus a few stops early and walk
Take the stairs instead of the elevator
Play with your children, don't just watch them play
Walk to the mailbox and skip the drive-through
Garden – rake the leaves, dig in the dirt, or mow the lawn
Dance around the house with your children or spouse
Clean the house – vacuum, wash windows, scrub floors
Go window-shopping – walk the mall
Contact your local recreation department for a schedule of exercise classes and a list of outdoor walking trails

---

All activity counts for health improvements such as managing stress, improving mood, enhancing sleep quality, and improving heart health. But when your goal is weight loss and improved body composition, exercise intensity and variety matter, too. A sound exercise program should include aerobic exercise, strength training and stretching. Be sure to begin with an intensity appropriate for your current fitness level and plan to add over-load, or gradually increase your exercise intensity, as your fitness level improves. The addition of over-load at appropriate intervals is the key to making continued progress toward your goal while avoiding over-use injuries and plateaus.

> *The CURVES signature 30- minute workout burns 184 calories and qualifies as moderate-intensity exercise, similar to a half-hour walk on the treadmill at 4mph, according to a recent study commissioned by the American Council on Exercise.*

Fitness for the Heart

Aerobic exercise is fitness training for the heart; it is often referred to as cardio because it improves the strength and efficiency of the heart. Aerobic exercise involves rhythmic, continuous movements of the large muscle groups, such as the legs, chest and back, over a sustained period of time. Activities like walking, jogging and swimming are aerobic and develop muscular endurance. You should include regular cardio exercise in your post-op lifestyle; the extra calories you burn will help you lose weight and improve your body composition. See Table 31.2 for examples and benefits of aerobic exercise. See Appendix I for sample cardio programs targeting a variety of fitness levels: beginners, intermediate & advanced.

Table 31.2
Benefits of and Examples of Activities that Are Aerobic

Benefits	*Aerobic Activities*
Burns calories	walking
Improves heart health	jogging
Improves mood	cycling (indoor or out)
Better hunger control	stair climbing
Eases stress	swimming
Improves body composition	step or dance aerobics
Everyday activities are easier	water aerobics

Power Up Your Weight Loss with Strength Training

You may not think of strength training as an essential component of your weight-loss program. But when you consider that your resting metabolic rate (RMR) increases as you add lean body mass (muscle), you can see the connection between lifting weights and staying trim. Because muscle tissue burns more calories, day and night, it takes more energy for your body to maintain muscle than it does to store fat. A challenge for anyone dieting to lose weight is that you'll lose lean body mass along with body fat. Although cardio helps you burn more calories, if you approach weight loss with diet and cardio alone, you lose muscle, too, which ultimately slows your metabolism.

People who have had weight loss surgery experience inevitable muscle losses during the rapid weight-loss phase immediately following surgery and throughout their weight-loss process. Also, the body's calorie burning engine naturally slows down with age. We lose an average of three to five percent of our lean body mass per decade after age thirty; this loss accelerates after age sixty-five. However, much of the muscle we lose during weight loss and with age can be blunted by staying active and doing strength training regularly.

As the years go by, you can put on body fat and increase a pant size or two, even though your body weight may stay the same. This occurs when compact muscle tissue is lost and the body's metabolism slows down, resulting in an increase in fluffier fat stores. Don't rely solely on the scale! Measure your body fat and include strength training in your fitness plan to maintain a healthy weight and body composition.

Finally, consider that lifting weights not only strengthens your muscles, but also builds the strength of your bones. The body constantly monitors the level of stress your muscles put on your bones. Low levels of stress signal the body to break down bone, whereas more stress signals the body to build bone.

Top 10 Reasons You Should Start Lifting Weights Today

10. *For a shapely physique.* More lean body mass improves the body's tone and firmness.
9. *To improve posture.* Weight training improves the way you hold your body and carry yourself.
8. *Protection from injury.* When you train your muscles you also improve the strength of your bones, tendons and ligaments.
7. *Greater confidence.* Meeting challenges in the weight room will give you an inner-strength that can carry into other areas of your life.
6. *Cardiovascular benefits* such as a strong, healthy heart, improved blood pressure and an increase in HDL cholesterol (the good cholesterol.)
5. *Strength train to make aerobic exercise easier.* By strengthening muscles and connective tissue with weights, you will find aerobic exercise more enjoyable and your goals more attainable.
4. *To reduce stress and improve your mood.*
3. *To become more independent.* Greater strength means everyday activities are easier.
2. *To maintain strong, healthy bones* and decrease your risk for bone fractures and osteoporosis.
1. *Meet and maintain your goal weight with ease.* Strength training keeps your calorie-burning engine revved up. More muscle = a higher metabolism!

You'll have stronger bones if you stay active and exercise regularly. Strength training, as well as weight bearing exercises like walking, jogging and aerobic dance, improves bone strength. However, exercise that does not require your bones to work against gravity, such as bicycling and swimming, does not build bone density.

> *Include weight training at least two days per week. Lean muscle helps keep your metabolism up, which means you'll burn more calories throughout the day.*

The time to start lifting weights is now. Whether you are completely sedentary or exercising regularly, in your twenties or in your seventies, increasing your muscle mass will result in immediate and long-term health benefits. See Appendix J and see our web-site at www.theroadtowlssuccess.com for sample resistance training programs and guidelines for getting started.

Flexibility

Age, exercise, and everyday activities such as sitting at our desks or behind a steering wheel result in tighter muscles. Over time we may notice our poor flexibility when simple movements like bending over to tie our shoes becomes a strain. The good news is it doesn't take a lot of time to improve your flexibility; the key is timing and consistency.

The best time to stretch is the last few minutes of your aerobic or strength workout, when your muscles are warm and pliable. Your muscles, like taffy, are resistant to stretch when cold, but easy to elongate when warm. So use flexibility training to close your workout sessions. Stretching feels great, it may alleviate some of your post-exercise muscle soreness and is a great time to relax and acknowledge your efforts. See Table 31.3 for a list of some of the benefits of stretching. Visit our web site at *www.theroadtowlssuccess.com* for pictures and detailed instructions on stretches for improving total body flexibility.

> *Flexibility training is the most over-looked component of fitness, yet it is essential for enhancing performance and decreasing your risk of injury.*

Yoga

I have been practicing and teaching yoga for several years now and I love it. It's hard for me to believe that I did not discover the gift of yoga earlier in life, which is why I want to share a little bit of information on it with you here.

Yoga is a word rooted in the Sanskrit language that literally means "to unite." The practice of yoga brings balance to body, mind and spirit by focusing on the inhalation and exhalation of the breath while moving through a sequence of postures. Techniques include extension and flexion movements to lengthen and balance the spine; stationary postures that build strength and flexibility; and breath work and meditation to calm and center the mind. Depending on the style of yoga you choose, you can achieve aerobic benefits, increased strength and improved flexibility all in one session *and* leave relaxed and refreshed. Unlike walking on a treadmill or taking an aerobics class, where you may be listening to music on your headphones, watching the daily news or chatting with a friend, yoga allows you to quiet the mind and turn your focus inward.

Table 31.3
Some of the Many Benefits of Stretching

Decrease risk of injury
Increase physical performance
Reduce muscle soreness after exercising
Promote spinal health and decrease risk of low back pain
Decrease risk of over-use injuries to common joints such as
    the shoulder, knee, hip, ankle, elbow and wrist.
Increase blood and oxygen flow to the joints
Improve balance
Improve neuromuscular coordination
Improve posture
Move with greater ease and fluidity
Relax and recharge

Table 31.4
Some of the Many Benefits of Yoga

Increased strength and endurance
Greater flexibility and balance
Reduced stress level
Enhanced body awareness
Improved sleep quality
Better posture and muscle tone
Enhanced memory and concentration
Improved mood and a greater sense of well being

One of the first discoveries I made when starting my yoga practice was that I was chronically sore and tired. In my attempt to be a good role model and practice what I preach, I found myself over-exercising and not getting enough rest. It took the introspection of yoga for me to recognize this and adjust my approach. Today I am spending less time exercising and enjoying an *improved* level of fitness, more energy and better health overall.

Several of my patients have shared stories on how yoga has helped them in other, more serious areas of their lives. Some people deal with high levels of stress or unmet emotional needs with behaviors such emotional eating, excessive alcohol consumption, compulsive shopping or over-filling their calendars to keep life in a constant state of chaos. These behaviors are all coping mechanisms that allow a person to deny or avoid dealing with the real issue. However, the first step toward making a behavior change is to recognize that there is a problem. If this resonates with you, yoga may be a useful tool to help you tap-in instead of tune-out, while improving your health and fitness level. Consider meeting with a counselor to assist you with setting short-term goals, working on appropriate behavior changes and enlisting a support system. See Table 31.5 for some of the many benefits of yoga. Visit our web sit at *www.theroadtowlssuccess.com* for a list of yoga resources and ideas for adding yoga to your lifestyle.

Overcoming Fitness Plateaus

Humans are creatures of habit. We resist change and prefer to stick with what's familiar. Think about it – we've all had that monotonous fitness experience; you know the one, where you always do the same thing. Whether it's thirty minutes on the treadmill, a familiar routine in the weight room, or the same workout at CURVES, there is little variety from day to day or month to month. What about the lady you have observed walking through your neighborhood consistently for the past year or more … or the man who seems to be at the gym every day of the week, yet he/she looks exactly the same? Yes, familiar fitness will ultimately result in a frustrating weight-loss standstill. However, with proper exercise planning, fitness plateaus can be minimized or completely avoided.

The principle of overload states that in order for a muscle, including the heart, to increase strength it must be gradually stressed by working against a load greater than it is used to. To increase muscular endurance, muscles must work for a longer period of time than they are used to. To improve muscular strength the amount of weight lifted, the number of repetitions lifted, and/or the number of sets completed must be increased. If the stress (exercise) is removed, there will be a decrease in fitness. If the amount of exercise stays the same, the current fitness level will be maintained.

Put simply, to avoid a stand-still with your fitness goals, mix things up a little bit! A tried and true approach to avoiding fitness plateaus is the F. I. T. approach. This acronym stands for: fitness, intensity and time. Increasing any one of these variables in your current program will accomplish overload and keep you moving toward your goal. See Table 31.5 for more on F. I. T. and how to apply this approach to your fitness program.

Table 31.5
The F. I. T. Approach to Avoiding Fitness Plateaus

Frequency: how often you exercise. – Example: walk 4 days per week instead of 3.

Intensity: a measure of difficulty or level of challenge you perceive from exercise. Example 1: Increase the treadmill incline or your walking or jogging speed to increase the intensity. Example 2: To increase the intensity of your resistance training program, increase the amount of weight you lift on a given exercise by less than or equal to 10%; or keep the weight lifted the same, but increase the number of sets performed, or the number of repetitions performed in eash set.

Note: the intensity of your exercise program should be specific to your current fitness level. The best way to measure your intensity when performing aerobic exercise is to monitor your heart rate. See Appendix K to learn how to calculate and use your personalized target heart rate range.

Time: how long you perform an activity. Time may also refer to the number of repetitions or sets completed when lifting weights. Example: walk for 40 minutes instead of 30 minutes – OR – complete 3 sets on each weight lifting exercise instead of 2 sets of each.

> *Goals are often poorly defined, ambiguous*
> *statements that almost ensure failure.*
> *Example:: "I want to lose weight."*
> *When setting goals, be specific and*
> *describe the behavior change.*
> *Example: "I intend to lose ten pounds over the next two*
> *months by walking five days per week, for 30-45 minutes,*
> *at 65-75% of my maximum target heart rate."*

Increasing Your Commitment to Exercise

Only one third of people who begin an exercise program are still exercising by the end of their first year. The good news is studies show that exercise adherence is much greater if a friend or family member is included in your plans to exercise. Good advice for all of us to heed is to find a workout buddy.

Working out with a partner creates accountability. When other life demands conflict with your plans to exercise, you may be likely to let yourself off the hook. But when someone else is counting on you, it's likely you'll make a little more effort to get there. One of the reasons programs like Weight Watchers and CURVES are successful is that they meet our need for accountability. Personal trainers and group exercise classes are also great ways to enlist the support of others.

Generally, when choosing a workout partner, consider someone who is eager and willing to make a commitment, and has a similar level of fitness and a compatible schedule. That's one reason dogs make the best workout partners; they don't mind working around your schedule or your fitness level, they are always eager to go, and they are a lot less expensive than a personal trainer!

> *Find a workout buddy! Research shows we are more likely to stick*
> *with an exercise program if we include someone else with a similar*
> *goal. Consider a neighbor, your significant other, a peer from*
> *work, your children, a group exercise class, a personal trainer, or*
> *even your dog. If someone else is counting on you, you're likely to*
> *make it a higher priority.*

Probably the best way to improve your exercise compliance is to keep it fun. Find something you enjoy and invite a friend to come along. Consider in-line skating, training for a 5K walk/run, joining an outdoor cycling group, snorkeling, taking a tennis or golf lesson or trying a new group exercise class. See Table 31.6 for tips on starting and staying with an exercise program.

"Having a support group is essential. Everyone might think that *WWW* stands for *World Wide Web* ... but for me and my exercise buddies, it stands for "Where was Wendy?" Because when I don't show up for class, I get e-mails that simply state **WWW** in the subject line. I then have to reply with my reasons for being absent and promise to show up for the next class!

This really helps me stay on track!"

- **Wendy Cunningham**
200 pound weight loss
Surgery date: June 2001

Post-Chapter Exercises:

- *Exercise One:* Commit to three daily behaviors that will add physical activity to your lifestyle (see Table 31.1 for ideas to get you started.)
- *Exercise Two:* Make a list of unhelpful behaviors that prevent you from exercising regularly. Now, create at least two solutions for each obstacle. Put your solutions in writing and keep them in a place you can refer to when feeling challenged.
- *Exercise Three:* Set two or three specific, short-term goals that you can start working on today.
- *Exercise Four:* Make a list of people you can count on for support and plan to lean on them regularly.
- *Exercise Five:* Consider which time of day is best for you to exercise and whether you are likely to be more compliant in a class setting, with a partner or on you own. Then act on those decisions!

- *Exercise Six:* Choose one aerobic workout in Appendix I to begin your exercise program or increase the intensity of your current program.
- *Exercise Seven:* Practice gauging the intensity of your aerobic work-outs this week applying your target heart rate. Use the information in Appendix K to calculate your personal target heart rate range.

Table 31.6

Tips for Getting Started and Sticking With It

- **Start small** – set short-term, realistic goals.
- **Keep it simple** – just do it!
- **Plan ahead** – schedule time for exercise.
- **Be consistent** – this creates positive momentum.
- **Make it a priority** – make an appointment for you.
- **Grab a partner** –create accountability.
- **Dress comfortably** – you *can* gain without pain.
- **Consider convenience** – exercise should lower your stress level not increase it.
- **Add variety** – use the F. I. T. approach.
- **Don't over-do-it** – no weekend warriors, please!
- **Get enough sleep** – rest is an important part of the equation.
- **Keep a good attitude** – focus on the positive.
- **Drink enough fluids** – even slight dehydration can zap your energy level.
- **Record your accomplishments** – keep a food and exercise diary.
- **Measure your progress** – schedule regular fitness assessments with your personal trainer or gym – seeing your positive results helps keep you going.
- **Make it a lifestyle** – there's no magic pill or quick fix. Take it one day at a time and enjoy the process.

Ten Tips to Keep You Motivated

◆ **Set short-term, realistic goals.** Then reward yourself for your successes with calorie-free treats like a massage, facial, manicure or pedicure.

◆ **Subscribe to a fitness magazine** for articles, pictures, recipes and ideas that inspire you.

◆ **Use a heart rate monitor.** You'll be less focused on the time and more likely to work at an appropriate intensity level.

◆ **Listen to music.** For a boost, play your favorite tunes on your iPod or headset.

◆ **Work out at the best time for you.** Figure out when your energy level is at its highest and get moving at that time.

◆ **Hire a trainer.** For your regular workouts, or just periodically. It will keep things new and fun!

◆ **Invest in comfortable, flattering workout clothes** that make you feel good about yourself.

◆ **Get over it!** Don't beat yourself up if you miss a workout. Focus on the ones you have done, and then get back on track.

◆ **Change the scenery.** If you do every workout at the gym, try doing a few outside if weather permits. Run the stadium steps instead of using the stair machine, do yoga at the park instead of in a class, ride your mountain bike instead of the stationary bike. Get creative.

◆ **Just do it!** Start your workout, even if you just feel lazy. Put on your workout clothes, tie your shoes, get out there and start moving. Chances are by the time you do all that your mind will be in the game.

Appendix A
Servings List for Meat and Other Protein-Rich Foods
(Fill Plate Section 1 with these foods)

<u>1 Serving = 7 grams of Protein.</u> In general, one meat serving is equivalent to 1 egg or 1 oz. of meat, fish, poultry or cheese.

List of Servings for Low-Fat Meat and Other Protein-Rich Foods:

Carbohydrate	*Protein*	*Fat*	*Calories*
0	7	0-4	35-55

<u>Food</u>

Serving Size Equivalent
<u>to 7 grams of Protein</u>

Beef
USDA Select or Choice grades of lean beef (trimmed of fat) such as round, sirloin and flank steak; tenderloin; roast (rib, chuck, rump); steak (T-bone, porterhouse, cubed); ground round .... 1 oz.

Cheese
Non-fat cheese...1 oz.
Skim or low-fat cottage cheese ....1/4 Cup
Grated Parmesan cheese ....2 Tbsp.
(or any variety of low-fat cheese with 4 grams or less fat/oz.)

Fish/Shellfish
Fresh or frozen cod, flounder, haddock, halibut, trout, tuna, herring, salmon, clams, lobster, scallops, shrimp .... 1 oz.
Oysters ....6 medium
Sardines ....2 medium

Game
Duck, pheasant, goose (no skin), venison, buffalo, ostrich, rabbit ....1 oz.

Lamb
Roast, chop, leg..1 oz.

Pork
Lean pork, such as fresh ham; canned, cured, or boiled ham; Canadian bacon; tenderloin ....1 oz.

Poultry
Chicken or turkey (white or dark meat, no skin), Cornish hen (no skin), domestic duck or goose (well-drained of fat, no skin)..1 oz.

Veal
Lean chop, roast...1 oz.

Other
Processed sandwich meats with 4 grams or less fat per ounce such as turkey, ham, roast beef..............................1 oz.
Egg whites..2
Egg Substitute, plain ....1/4 Cup
Hot dogs with 4 grams of fat or less per ounce ......1.5 oz.
Sausage with 4 grams of fat or less per oune. ....1 oz.
Liver, kidney, heart (high in cholesterol)................1 oz.

List of Servings for Medium-to-High--Fat Meat and Other Protein-Rich Foods:

List of Servings for Low-Fat Meat and Other Protein-Rich Foods:			
Carbohydrate	*Protein*	*Fat*	*Calories*
0	7	5-8	75-100

Food

Serving Size Equivalent to 7 grams of Protein

Beef
Most beef products fall into this category. Ground beef, meatloaf, corned beef, short ribs and prime grades of meat trimmed of fat (e.g. prime rib)..............................1 oz.

Cheese
(5 grams of fat or less per ounce):
Feta..1 oz.
Mozzarella...1 oz.
Ricotta..1/4 Cup
(8 grams of fat or less per ounce):
American ....1 oz.
Cheddar..1 oz.
Monterey Jack ....1 oz.
Swiss ....1 oz.

Fish
Any fried fish product ....1 oz.

Lamb
Rib roast or ground..1 oz.

Pork
Top loin, chop, Boston butt, cutlet, spareribs, ground pork, pork sausage .... 1 oz.

Poultry
Chicken (dark meat with skin), ground turkey or ground chicken, fried chicken (with skin) .... 1 oz.

Veal
Cutlet (ground or cubed, unbreaded) .... 1 oz.

Other
Processed sandwich meats such as bologna and pimento loaf (8 grams of fat or less per serving) .... 1 oz.
Sausage, such as bratwurst, Italian, knockwurst, Polish, smoked .... 1 oz.
Hot dog .... 1.5 oz.
Bacon .... 3 Slices
Peanut Buter .... 2 Tbsp.

Appendix B

Servings List for Non-Starchy Vegetables

(Fill Plate Section 2 with these Vegetables)

1 Serving = 5 grams of Carbohydrate

1 Serving = ½ Cup Cooked or 1 Cup un-cooked
of any of the following vegetables:

Artichoke

Mushrooms

Asparagus

Beans (green, wax, Italian)

Bean sprouts

Beets

Broccoli

Brussels Sprouts

Cabbage

Carrots

Cauliflower

Celery

Collard Greens

Cucumber

Eggplant

Green onions or Scallions

Kale

Kohlrabi

Leeks

Mustard Greens

Okra

Onions

Pea Pods

Peppers (all varieties)

Radishes

Salad Greens (all varieties)

Sauerkraut

Spinach

Tomatoes, fresh or canned

Turnips

Water Chestnuts

Watercress

Zucchini

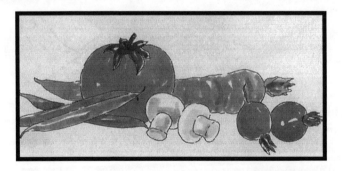

Appendix C
Servings List for High Carbohydrate, Starchy Foods
(Choose these foods last to fill plate section 3.
Do not exceed 30 grams of total carbohydrate between
section 2 and section 3 of your plate at each meal.)

High Carbohydrate foods include all fruit, starchy
vegetables, bread, cereal and other grain products.
1 Serving = 15 grams of Carbohydrate/Starch

Starchy Vegetables

Food	Serving Size Equivalent to 15 grams of Carbohydrates
Baked beans	1/3 Cup
Corn	1/2 Cup
Corn on cob, medium	1 (5 oz.)
Mixed vegetables with corn,peas or pasta	1 Cup
Peas, green	1/2 Cup
Plantain	1/2 Cup
Potato, baked or boiled	1 small
Potato, mashed	1/2 Cup
Squash, winter (acorn, butternut, pumpkin	1 Cup
Yam, sweet potato, plain	1/2 Cup

High-Protein-Starchy-Vegetables
(Count as 1 starch serving plus 1 low-fat protein serving)

Food	Serving Size Equivalent to 15 grams of Carbohydrates
Beans and peas (garbanzo, pinto, kidney, black-eyed, split, white)	1/2 Cup
Lima beans	2/3 Cup
Lentils	1/2 Cup
Miso	3 Tbsp.

Fruit

Food	Serving Size Equivalent to 15 grams of Carbohydrates
Apple, unpeeled, small	1 (4 oz.)
Applesauce, unsweetened	½ Cup
Apples, dried	4 rings
Apricots, fresh	4 whole (5.5 oz.)
Apricots, dried	8 halves
Banana, small	1 (4 oz.)
Blackberies	¾ Cup
Blueberries	¾ Cup
Cantaloupe, small	½ melon (11 oz.) or 1 Cup cubes
Cherries, sweet, fresh	12 (3 oz.)
Cherries, sweet, canned	½ Cup
Dates	3 medium
Figs, fresh	2 medium
Fruit Cocktail	½ Cup
Grapefruit, large	½ (11 oz.)
Grapefruit sections, canned	¾ Cup
Grapes, small	17 (3 oz.)
Honeydew melon	1 slice (10 oz.) or 1 Cup cubes
Kiwi	1 (3.5 oz.)
Mandarin Oranges, canned	¾ Cup
Mango, small	½ fruit (5.5 oz.) or ½ Cup
Nectarine, small	1 (5 oz.)
Orange, small	1 (6.5 oz.)
Papaya	1.2 fruit (5.5 oz.) or ½ Cup
Peach, medium, fresh	1 (6 oz.)
Peaches, canned	½ Cup

Pear, large, fresh ....½ (4 oz.)
Pears, canned ....½ Cup
Pineapple, fresh ....¾ Cup
Pineapple, canned ....½ Cup
Plums, small ....2 (5 oz.)
Plums, canned ....½ Cup
Prunes, dried ....3 medium
Raisins ....2 Tbsp.
Raspberries ....1 Cup
Strawberries ....1 ¼ Cup of
....whole berries
Tangerines, small ....2 (8 oz.)
Watermelon ....1 Slice (13.5 oz.)
.... or 1 ¼ Cup cubes

Common Measurements

3 Tsp. = 1 Tbsp.   4 ounces = ½ Cup
4 Tbsp. = ¼ Cup   8 ounces = 1 Cup
5 1/3 Tbsp. = 1/3 Cup   1 Cup = ½ Pint

Bread, Cereals and Grains

	Serving Size Equivalent
Food	to 15 grams of Carbohydrates

Bagel ....1/2 (1 oz.)
Bread, reduced-calorie ....2 Slices (1.5 oz.)
Bread (white, wheat, pumpernickel, rye).......1 Slice
Bread sticks, crisp, 4 in. long X ½ in 2
English muffin 1/2
Hot dog or hamburger bun ....1/2 (1 oz.)
Pita, 6 in. across 1/2
Raisin bread, unfrosted ....1 Slice (1 oz.)

Roll, plain, small ....1 (1 oz.)
Tortilla, corn, 6 in. across..........................1
Tortilla, flour, 6 in. across..........................1
Waffle, 4 ½ in. square, reduced fat ....3 Tbsp.
Bran Cereal ....1/2 Cup
Bulgur...1/2 Cup
Cereal, sweet ....1/2 Cup
Cereal, unsweet...3/4 Cup
Cornmeal (dry) ....3 Tbsp.
Couscous ....1/3 Cup
Flour (dry) ....3 Tbsp.
Granola, low-fat ....1/4 Cup
Grape Nuts ....1/4 Cup
Grits...1/2 Cup
Kasha..1/2 Cup
Millet..1/4 Cup
Muesli...1/4 Cup
Oats ....1/2 Cup
Pasta...1 Cup
Puffed cereal ....1 ½ Cups
Rice Milk..1/2 Cup
Rice, white or brown ....1/3 Cup
Shredded Wheat..1/2 Cup
Sugar-frosted cereal ....1/2 Cup
Wheat germ ....3 Tbsp.

Crackers and Snacks

	Serving Size Equivalent
Food	to 15 grams of Carbohydrates

Animal Crackers 8
Graham crackers, 2 ½ in. square 3
Matzoh ....3/4 oz.
Melba toast ....4 Slices
Oyster crackers..24
Popcorn (popped, no-fat-added) ....3 Cups
Pretzels..3/4 oz.
Rice cakes, 4 in. across 2
Saltine-type crackers....................................6
Snack chips, fat-free (tortilla, potato)...........15-20 (3/4 oz.)
Whole-wheat crackers, no fat added ....3-5 (3/4 oz.)

Starchy Foods Prepared with Fat
(Count as 1 serving of starch plus 5 grams of fat)

	Serving Size Equivalent
Food	to 15 grams of Carbohydrates

Biscuit, 2 ½ in. across 1
Chow mein noodles ....1/2 Cup
Corn bread, 2 in. cube ....1 (2 oz.)
Crackers, round butter type..........................6
Croutons...1 Cup
French-fried potatoes....................................16-25 (3 oz.)
Granola...1/4 Cup
Muffin, small ....1 (1.5 oz.)
Pancake, 4 in. across.....................................2
Popcorn, microwave ....3 Cups
Sandwich crackers (cheese or
peanut butter filling) 3

Stuffing, bread (prepared).............................1/3 Cup
Taco shell, 6 in. across.................................2
Waffle, 4 ½ in. square 1
Whole-wheat crackers, fat added ....4-6 (1 oz.)

Starches that Swell When Cooked

Food	Serving Size Equivalent to 15 grams of Carbohydrate	
	Uncooked	**Cooked**
Oatmeal	3 Tbsp.	½ Cup
Cream of Wheat	2 Tbsp.	½ Cup
Grits	3 Tbsp.	½ Cup
Rice	2 Tbsp.	1/3 Cup
Spaghetti	¼ Cup	½ Cup
Noodles	1/3 Cup	½ Cup
Macaroni	¼ Cup	½ Cup
Dried beans or peas	¼ Cup	½ Cup
Lentils	3 Tbsp.	½ Cup

Fat-Free and Low-Fat Milk and Yogurt
(Count as 1 starch serving and 1 protein serving)

Food	Serving Size Equivalent to 15 grams of Carbohydrate

Fat-free milk...1 Cup
1/2% milk...1 Cup
1% milk ....1 Cup
Fat-free or low-fat buttermilk.......................1 Cup
Evaporated fat-free milk ....1/2 Cup
Fat-free dry milk ....1/3 Cup, dry
Plain non-fat yogurt ....3/4 Cup
Sweetened-fruit-flavored, non-fat yogurt.......1/3 Cup
Non-fat or low-fat fruit-flavored yogurt
sweetened with sugar substitute...................1 Cup

Reduced Fat and Yogurt

(Count as 1 starch serving, 1 protein serving plus 5 grams of fat)

Food	Serving Size Equivalent to 15 grams of Carbohydrate
2 % milk	1 Cup
Plain low-fat yogurt	3/4 Cup
Sweetened-fruit-flavored yogurt with fat	1/3 Cup
Sweet acidophilus milk	1 Cup

Whole Milk

(Count as 1 starch serving, 1 protein serving plus 8 grams of fat)

Food	Serving Size Equivalent to 15 grams of Carbohydrate
Whole milk	1 Cup
Evaporated whole milk	1/2 Cup
Goat's milk	1 Cup
Kefir	1 Cup

Appendix D

The New Food Guide Pyramid

The government's new Food Guide Pyramid offers more personal guidelines based on your age, gender and activity level. To take advantage of the many consumer-friendly tools, visit: www.mypyramid.gov.

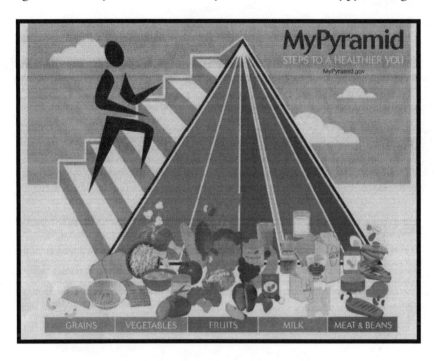

Appendix E
A Guide for Satisfying Your Sweet Tooth

	Saccharin	Aspartame
Products & Brands	Sweet 'N Low Sugar Twin Necta Sweet Hermesteas	NutraSweet Equal
FDA Approved	As a table-top sweetener in foods & as a sweetener in beverages, not to exceed 12 mg/fl. oz.	As a general purpose sweetener for use in all foods & beverages since 1996
Compared to Sugar	200 to 700 times sweeter	160 to 220 times sweeter
Acceptable Daily Intake	5 mg/kg body weight	50 mg/kg of body weight
Product Characteristics	Equivalent to the sweetening power of 1 tsp. of sugar	1 packet (35-50 mg of aspartame) is the equivalent sweetness of 2 tsp. of sugar
Nutrition & Health	No evidence based data supporting it is carcinogenic	Phenylketonuria (PKU) sufferers should be cautious.
When used for Cooking	Maintains its sweet flavor when heated, may not be suitable in all recipes because it has less bulk than sugar.	Loses sweetness with prolonged exposure to high temperatures; add toward the end of cooking to preserve sweet taste.

Acesulfame-K	Sucralose	Stevia
Sunett Sweet One	Splenda	Stevia
As a general purpose sweetener since 1988	As a general purpose sweetener since 1999	Not approved for use as a food additive; may be used as a dietary supplement.
Approximately 200 times sweeter	600 times sweeter	250 to 300 times sweeter
Has a high degree of stability over a wide range of pH and temperature storage conditions	The only non-caloric sweetener created from sucrose	A natural sweetener derived from a plant extract
95 percent of consumed sweetener is excreted in urine and thus, does not provide energy	Chemically modified to become a non-nutritive powder so the body does not recognize it as a carbohydrate	A natural sweetener with no calories
Can withstand high cooking and baking temperatures. Sweetening power is not reduced with heating. It does not give bulk or volume, so it may not be suitable for all recipes.	Sweetening power is not reduced with heating. Doesn't give bulk to baked goods, but is heat stable in cooking and baking.	Stevia is acid and heat stable up to 200 degrees Celsius. Stevia does not add texture, caramelize, enhance browning, help soften butter, nor aid yeast fermentation as sugar does in baking.

4 - Week Sample Meal Plan

Appendix F
Week One

Day One

Breakfast	Plate Section #	Food Source	Grams
Egg, Cheese & Ham Omelet			
2 Whole Eggs (or ½ Cup Egg Replacement)	1	Protein	14g
1 oz. of Cheese	1	Protein	7g
1 oz. of Deli Ham (or other meat variety)	1	Protein	7g
1 Slice of Toast* OR 1 Serving of Fruit**	3	Carb.	15g

Lunch
Tuna Salad			
3 oz. of water-packed Tuna on top of:	1	Protein	21g
1 Cup Salad Greens	2	Carb.	5g
1-2 Tbsp. Salad Dressing (any variety) OR	--	Fat	5-10g
2 Tbsp. Light Mayonnaise + relish to taste	--	Fat	5-10g
10 Crackers OR 1 Slice of Bread	3	Carb.	15-20g

Dinner
3 oz. Grilled Salmon with Rosemary (see Recipe)	1	Protein	21g
1 Cup Steamed Asparagus	2	Carb.	10g
1/3 Cup Rice	3	Carb.	15g

Day Two

Breakfast
Bacon, Egg & Cheese Sandwich			
1 Whole Egg (or ¼ Cup Egg Substitute)	1	Protein	7g
2 Slices of Canadian Bacon	1	Protein	7g
¼ Cup Grated Cheddar Cheese (1 oz.)	1	Protein	7g
1 – 2 Slices of Fresh Tomato	2	Carb.	3g
½ Bagel (or 20 grams of Carbohydrate)	3	Carb	20g

Lunch
Ham & Cheese Sandwich			
2 oz. of Ham	1	Protein	14g
1 oz. of Cheese	1	Protein	7g
1 Slice of Tomato & Lettuce	2	Carb.	5g
2 Slices of Low Carb Bread*	3	Carb.	22g
Mustard, Light Mayo or Pepper to taste	--		

Dinner
3 oz. Orange Roughy in Ginger Sauce (see Recipe)	1	Protein	21g
1 Cup Steamed Snow Peas	2	Carb.	10g
1/3 Cup Brown Rice	3	Carb.	15g

Day Three

Breakfast	Plate Section #	Food Source	Grams
Scrambled Eggs (1 egg + ¼ Cup egg substitute)	1	Protein	14g
1 Yogurt (10 grams of Carb or less)	1 & 3	Protein+Carb	7g/10g
1–2 Tbsp. Texturized Soy Protein* (sprinkled on top of yogurt)	1	Protein	5 g

Lunch

Grilled-Cheese Sandwich			
2 Slices of Low Carb Bread*	3	Carb.	22g
2 oz. of Cheese	1	Protein	14g
¼ Cup Peanuts	1	Protein	7g

Dinner

3 oz. Grilled Mahi Mahi	1	Protein	21g
1 Cup Steamed Spinach	2	Carb.	10g
½ Cup Baked Potato Fries	3	Carb.	15g

* Texturized Soy (or Vegetable) Protein or TVP can be found in health food or specialty grocery stores and is a good source of protein that is low in carbohydrate.

Day Four

Breakfast

Cheese Toast + A Side of Eggs

2 Slices of Low Carbohydrate Bread*	3	Carb.	22g
2 oz. of Cheese (any variety)	1	Protein	14g
1-2 Eggs (any variety)	1	Protein	7-14g

Lunch

Egg Salad Sandwich

2 - 3 Boiled Eggs	1	Protein	14-21g
1 – 2 Tbsp. Light Mayo	--	Fat	10-15g
Pepper to taste --	--	--	
1 – 2 Slices of Low Carb Bread*	3	Carb.	11-22g

Dinner

Chicken and Vegetable Kabobs with Cucumber-Vinegar Salad

3 oz. of Grilled Chicken Breast	1	Protein	21g
½ Red Bell Pepper	2	Carb.	5g
½ Yellow Bell Pepper	2	Carb.	5g
½ Onion	2	Carb.	5g
½ Sliced Cucumber with Oil and Vinegar	2	Carb.	5g

Day Five

Breakfast	Plate Section #	Food Source	Grams
1 Apple**	3	Carb.	15g
2 Tbsp. Peanut or Almond Butter	1	Protein/Fat	8g/16g
2 oz. Cheese	1	Protein	14g

Lunch

	Plate Section #	Food Source	Grams
Reuben Sandwich 2 Slices of Low Carb Rye Bread*	3	Carb.	22g
2 oz. of Corned Beef	1	Protein	14g
1 oz. of Cheese	1	Protein	7g
2 Tbsp. Sauerkraut	2	Carb.	5g

Dinner

	Plate Section #	Food Source	Grams
3 oz. of Baked Chicken Breast	1	Protein	21g
1 Cup Green Beans with Sliced Almonds	2	Carb.	10g
Tossed Salad (mixed greens, cucumbers, tomatoes)	2	Carb.	5g
1-2 Tbsp. Salad Dressing (any variety)***	--	Fat	10-15g

Day Six

Breakfast

	Plate Section #	Food Source	Grams
Scrambled Eggs (½ Cup Egg Substitute)	1	Protein	14g
1 Slice Canadian Bacon	1	Protein	7g
1 Serving of Fruit (any variety)**	3	Carb.	15 g

Lunch

	Plate Section #	Food Source	Grams
Grilled Chicken Salad			
3 oz. Chicken Breast	1	Protein	21g
1 Cup Salad Greens	2	Carb.	10g
1-2 Tbsp. Salad Dressing	--	Fat	10-15g
1 small roll	3	Carb.	15g

Dinner

	Plate Section #	Food Source	Grams
3 oz. Grilled New York Strip	1	Protein	21g
1 Cup Steamed Broccoli	2	Carb.	10g
1/3 Cup Baked Beans	3	Carb.	15g

Day Seven

Breakfast	Plate Section #	Food Source	Grams
French Toast with a Side of Bacon			
2 Slices of Low Carbohydrate Bread*	3	Carb.	22g
½ Cup Egg Substitute	1	Protein	14g
3 Slices of Bacon	1	Protein	7g

Lunch

	Plate Section #	Food Source	Grams
PB&J Sandwich with a Side of Cheese			
2 Slices of Low-Carb Bread*	3	Carb.	22g
1 Heaping Tbsp. of Peanut Butter	1	Protein	4g
1 tsp. of Low Carb Jelly	3	Carb.	2g
1-2 oz. of Low Fat Cheese	1	Protein	7-14g

Dinner

	Plate Section #	Food Source	Grams
3 oz. of Ginger-Chicken Breast (152)	1	Protein	21g
1 Cup Steamed Green Beans	2	Carb.	10g
1 Cup Mandarin Orange-Vinaigrette Salad	2	Carb.	15g

* Low Carbohydrate Bread = less than or equal to 11 grams of Carbohydrate per slice. Feel free to choose a higher carbohydrate bread and reduce your serving size to keep your total grams of carbohydrate within your budget at each meal.

** One Fruit Serving = 15 grams of Carbohydrate; See Fruit Exchanges in Appendix C

*** Salad Dressing does not need to be Fat-Free; try to limit the grams of fat in the entire meal to 15 grams total. Also, note that some salad dressing(s) can be a hidden source of carbohydrate.

Recipes

Week One

Grilled Salmon with Rosemary: Serves 4
1 pound salmon
1 Tbsp. olive oil
2 tsp. lemon juice
¼ tsp. salt
¼ tsp. pepper
2 cloves of garlic
2 tsp. rosemary leaves or 1 tsp. dried rosemary

Cut salmon into four equal-portions. Combine the olive oil, lemon juice, salt, pepper, garlic and rosemary in a bowl. Brush the mixture onto the fish and cook over medium heat to an internal temperature of 140 degrees Fahrenheit (approximately 4-6 minutes per ½ inch meat thickness; if meat is more than one inch thick, gently turn it half-way through grilling.

Nutrition At A Glance: Per Serving
Protein: 23 grams
Carbohydrate: 1 gram
Fat: 3 grams

Gingered-Orange Roughy: Serves 4
2/3 Cup dry Sherry or Vermouth
1/3 Cup low-sodium soy sauce
1 Tbsp. Sesame Oil
½ Cup finely chopped green onion
2 tsp. freshly grated ginger
2 tsp. finely chopped garlic
4 orange roughly fillets

Preheat the oven to 400 degrees Fahrenheit. Mix the sherry or vermouth, soy sauce, sesame oil, onion, ginger and garlic in a small bowl. Place the fish fillets in an oven-safe dish and drizzle the marinade over the fish. Bake for 12 minutes or until fish flakes easily.

Grilled Chicken Breast with Ginger: Serves 4

1 Tbsp. lemon juice
1 ½ tsp. grated fresh ginger
½ tsp. freshly ground black pepper
2 cloves of garlic
4 split chicken breasts (cook with skin, then remove)

Combine the lemon juice, ginger, pepper and garlic in a small bowl. Place the chicken breasts in a deep bowl. Pour the ginger mixture over the breasts, turning once to coat both sides. Cover and refrigerate for 30 minutes to 2 hours. Grill the chicken to an internal temperature of 160 degrees Fahrenheit. Place the chicken breasts on a platter and cover with foil for five minutes; this will allow the internal meat temperature to rise to a minimum of 165 degrees Fahrenheit. Remove the chicken skin and serve immediately.

Mandarin Orange-Vinaigrette Salad: Serves 2

2 Cups Mixed Salad Greens
1 Cup Mandarin Oranges (fresh or canned)
½ Cup Dates (chopped)
¼ Cup Vinaigrette Salad Dressing

Pour salad dressing over mixed greens and toss to coat. Top greens with dates and oranges. Serve.

Week Two

Day One

Breakfast	Plate Section #	Food Source	Grams
2 hard-boiled eggs	1	Protein	14g
1 oz. Cheese (any variety)	1	Protein	7g
1 Slice Low Carb Toast	1	Carb.	11g
½ Cup Blueberries	3	Carb.	15g

Lunch
Turkey & Cheese Roll-Ups with a Side of Fruit

	Plate Section #	Food Source	Grams
3 Slices of Turkey Breast	1	Protein	21g
1.5 oz. of Cheese (any variety)	1	Protein	10g
3 Medium Lettuce Leaves (any variety)	2	Carb.	3g
3-4 Tbsp. chopped tomato	2	Carb.	3g
Light Mayo, Mustard and/or Pepper to taste	--	--	--
1 Small Apple + 10 grapes (or 1½ Fruit Servings)	3	Carb.	2g

Dinner

	Plate Section #	Food Source	Grams
Meat Loaf – 2 Servings (See Recipe)	1	Protein	24g
½ Cup Steamed Asparagus	2	Carb.	5g

Day Two

Breakfast
Sunny-Side Up English Muffin with Fruit

	Plate Section #	Food Source	Grams
½ English Muffin	3	Carb.	15g
1 poached Egg	1	Protein	7g
1 oz. Cheese (any variety)	1	Protein	7g
1 Slice Canadian Bacon	1	Protein	6g
½ Medium Grapefruit	3	Carb.	10g

Lunch

	Plate Section #	Food Source	Grams
¾ Cup Low-Fat Cottage Cheese	1	Protein	21g
10 Crackers (20 grams of Carbohydrate)	3	Carb.	20g
1 Celery Stalk	2	Carb.	3g
1 Tbsp. Peanut Butter	1	Protein/Fat	4g/8g

Dinner

	Plate Section #	Food Source	Grams
3 oz. Roast Beef	1	Protein	21g
¾ Cup Steamed Carrots	2	Carb.	8g
3 Small Red Boiled Potatoes	3	Carb.	15g

Day Three

Breakfast	Plate Section #	Food Source	Grams
Egg White Omelette			
½ Cup Egg Substitute	1	Protein	12g
1 oz. Cheese (any variety)	1	Protein	7g
1 oz. ham/turkey/bacon	1	Protein	7g
1 Slice Low Carbohydrate Bread	3	Carb.	15g
½ Small Apple	3	Carb.	8 g

Lunch

	Plate Section #	Food Source	Grams
Apple Walnut Chicken Salad – 1 Serving (see Recipe)	1	Protein	27g

Dinner

	Plate Section #	Food Source	Grams
3 oz. Marinated Flank Steak	1	Protein	21g
1 Cup Green and Yellow Wax Beans	2	Carb.	10g
1 Slice Toasted Whole Grain Roll	3	Carb.	15g

Day Four

Breakfast

	Plate Section #	Food Source	Grams
1 Oatmeal Pancake (see Recipe)	1&3	Protein/Carb	28/30g

Lunch

	Plate Section #	Food Source	Grams
One 6-inch Pita filled with	3	Carb.	15g
3 oz. Sliced Turkey	1	Protein	21g
3 Tomato Slices	2	Carb.	2g
½ Cup Shredded Letuce	2	Carb.	3g
1 oz. Cheese (any variety)	1	Protein	6g
2 Tbsp. Salsa	2	Carb.	5g

Dinner

	Plate Section #	Food Source	Grams
3 oz. Grilled Salmon	1	Protein	21g
1 Cup Steamed Broccoli	2	Carb.	10g
1/3 Cup Couscous	3	Carb.	15g

Day Five

Breakfast	Plate Section #	Food Source	Grams
Sunrise Soyprise (see Recipe)	1&3	Protein/Carb.	22g/22g

Lunch
Chicken-Raspberry-Walnut Spinach Salad

	Plate Section #	Food Source	Grams
1 Cup Fresh Spinach Leaves topped with	2	Carb.	5g
3 oz. Grilled Chicken Breast	1	Protein	21g
1/3 Cup Fresh Raspberries	3	Carb.	5g
2 Tbsp. Chopped Walnuts	--	Fat	10g
1 Tbsp. Vinaigrette Salad Dressing	--	Fat	5g
1 Slice Whole Grain Bread or Crackers	3	Carb.	15g

Dinner

	Plate Section #	Food Source	Grams
Cumin Pork Loin with Dried Fruit (see Recipe)	1&3	Protein/Carb.	28g/13g
½ Cup Steamed Asparagus	2	Carb.	5g

Day Six

Breakfast

	Plate Section #	Food Source	Grams
¾ Cup Pineapple (fresh or canned)	3	Carb.	15g
¾ Cup 1% Cottage Cheese	1	Protein	21g
12 Almonds	--	Fat	10g

Lunch
Tuna Salad

	Plate Section #	Food Source	Grams
3 oz. of Water-Packed Tuna	1	Protein	21g
1 Tbsp. Mayonnaise (reduced fat)	--	Fat	5g
1 Tbsp. Celery (chopped)	2	Carb.	--
3-4 Slices Fresh Tomato	2	Carb.	3g
1 Cup Mixed Salad Greens	2	Carb.	5g
2 Tbsp. Walnuts (chopped)	--	Fat	10g
1 Slice Whole Grain Bread or 6-10 Crackers	3	Carb.	15g

Dinner

	Plate Section #	Food Source	Grams
Taco Salad (see Recipe)	1,2&3	Pro/Carb/Fat	30g/25g/15g

Day Seven

Breakfast	Plate Section #	Food Source	Grams
Scrambled Eggs (1 egg + ½ Cup egg substitute)	1	Protein	21g
½ Cup Shredded Wheat Cereal	3	Carb.	20g
½ Cup Skim Milk	3	Carb.	6g

Lunch

	Plate Section #	Food Source	Grams
Roasted Beef Wrap (see Recipe)	1,2&3	Pro/Carb/Fat	21g/ 25g/8g
12 Almonds	1	Pro/Fat	5g/5g

Dinner

	Plate Section #	Food Source	Grams
Stir-Fry Chicken & Vegetables	1 & 2	Pro/Carb	23g/10g
1/3 Cup Rice	3	Carb.	15 g

Recipes

Week Two

Meat Loaf: Serves 8
6 oz. of tomato paste (low sodium)
½ Cup dry red wine
½ Cup water
1 clover garlic, finely chopped
½ teaspoon basil (dried leaves)
¼ teaspoon oregano (dried leaves)
¼ teaspoon low-sodium salt
16 oz. ground turkey breast
1 Cup oatmeal
¼ Cup liquid egg substitute
½ Cup shredded zucchini

Preheat the oven to 350 degrees Fahrenheit. Combine tomato paste, wine, water, garlic, basil, oregano and salt in a small pan. Bring to a boil, then reduce the heat to low. Simmer, uncovered for 15 minutes. Set aside.

Combine the turkey, oatmeal, egg substitute, zucchini, and ½ Cup of tomato mixture in a large bowl. Mix well. Shape into a loaf and place into an un-greased loaf pan (8" x 4".) Bake for 45 minutes; drain off drippings. Pour ½ Cup of remaining tomato mixture on-top of the loaf. Bake for 15 additional minutes. Cool for 10 minutes and serve.

Nutrition At A Glance: Per Serving
Protein: 24 grams
Carbohydrate: 24 gram
Fat: 18 gram

Apple-Walnut Chicken Salad: Serves 2
6 oz. cooked chicken breast (cut into ½ inch cubes)
½ Cup chopped celery
½ Cup chopped apple
½ Cup chopped walnuts
1 Tbsp. raisins
4 Tbsp. Italian dressing

In medium bowl combine chicken, celery, apple, walnuts and raisins. Serve over 1 Cup mixed salad greens and top with Italian dressing.

Oatmeal Pancake: Serves 1

½ Cup quick-cook oatmeal
¼ Cup low-fat cottage cheese (or Tofu)
1 Cup egg substitute
1 tsp. vanilla extract
¼ tsp. cinnamon
¼ tsp. nutmeg

Combine oatmeal, cottage cheese, egg substitute, vanilla extract, cinnamon and nutmeg in a blender; process until smooth. Spray non-stick skillet with cooking spray. Add batter and cook both sides until lightly browned. Top with Splenda, Stevia or other non-calorie sugar substitute.

Nutrition At A Glance: Per Serving
Protein: 28 grams
Carbohydrate: 30 grams
Fat: 4 grams

Sunrise Soyprise: Serves 1

1 Cup light yogurt
(less than or equal to 15 g Total Carb)
2/3 Cup texturized soy protein
2 Tbsp. chopped almonds (or other nut of your choice)
2 Tbsp. sliced strawberries (or other berry of your choice)

Layer the yogurt and soy protein in a long-stem dessert glass. Top with chopped almonds and berries. Serve.

Nutrition At A Glance: Per Serving
Protein: 24 grams
Carbohydrate: 25 gram
Fat: 3 gram

Cumin Pork Loin with Dried Fruit: Serves 4

1 pound boneless pork loin
½ Cup mixed dried fruit (chopped)
¾ tsp. ground cumin
¼ tsp. salt
¼ tsp. salt
A small roasting pan
Kitchen string

Heat oven to 375 degrees Fahrenheit. Soak fruit in 1 Cup boiling water for 15 minutes. Make a long cut down the center of the pork loin approximately 2/3 deep (do not cut all the way through the meat.) Open meat like a book. Mix cumin, salt and pepper and spring ½ tsp. of mixture over cut surface of meat. Drain fruit; save liquid. Arrange fruit along the interior cut of meat. Tie in several places to close. Rub meat with remaining cumin mixture. Place in pan. Roast for 50 minutes or until meat thermometer registers 145 degrees Fahrenheit when inserted in the center of the meat. While meat cooks, add fruit liquid to pan and stir over high heat to dissolve browned bits on bottom. Simmer 4 minutes to reduce slightly. Serve over pork.

Nutrition At A Glance: Per Serving
Protein: 28 grams
Carbohydrate: 13 grams
Fat: 15 grams

Taco Salad: Serves 4

12 oz. lean ground beef or turkey
1 packet (1.25 oz.) taco seasoning mix (low sodium)
½ Cup kidney beans (canned and rinsed)
1 Cup salsa
4 Cups mixed salad greens
1 Cup fresh tomatoes, chopped
½ Cup cheddar cheese, shredded
¼ Cup red onion, chopped
1 bag corn tortilla chips

Heat a large non-stick skillet over medium-high heat. Add ground beef or turkey and cook, breaking up clumps with a wooden spoon, about 3 minutes or until no longer pink. Add taco seasoning, stir and cook another 1 minute. Stir in kidney beans and heat through. Place or break-up a hand-full of tortilla chips in 4 individual salad bowls (approximately 12 chips per bowl.) Cover chips with 1 Cup salad greens, 3 oz. of meat mixture and top with salsa, tomatoes, red onion and chips to taste.

Roasted Beef Wrap: Serves 1
1 Flour tortilla (8-10")
1 Tbsp. Cream cheese (reduced fat)
2 Tbsp. Red Onion
1/3 Cup fresh spinach leaves
3 oz. Roast beef

Spread cream cheese evenly over one-side of tortilla. Layer onion, spinach and roast beef on top. Fold or roll-up and serve.

Stir-Fry Chicken and Vegetables: Serves 4
3 Tbsp. Olive or Canola Oil
4 Cooked, Bone-less, Skin-less Chicken Breast (cut into 1/8th inch strips)
10 oz. of frozen non-starchy vegetables (e.g. broccoli, green beans, red bell peppers and mushrooms)
2 Tbsp. Water
2 Tbsp. Soy Sauce (reduced sodium)
10 oz. Fresh Spinach

Heat skillet or wok over high heat. Add 1 ½ Tbsp. of oil and gently rotate pan to coat surface. Add chicken and stir-fry for 2 minutes. Remove chicken to a bowl. Add remaining oil to skillet and coat the surface. Add vegetables and stir-fry for about 4 minutes. Return chicken to skillet. Add water and soy sauce and stir-fry for 2 minutes. Add spinach. Cover the pan and steam over medium heat for 2 minutes. Gently turn the spinach leaves once, using a tongs; cover and steam another 2 minutes. Serve chicken and vegetables on top or with a side of rice.

Week Three

Day One

Breakfast	Plate Section #	Food Source	Grams
½ Cup Oatmeal (cooked)	3	Carb.	15g
½ Banana, Small	3	Carb.	7g
Scrambled Eggs (1 whole egg + ½ Cup Egg Substitute)	1	Protein	21g

Lunch
Open Face PB & J Sandwich w/ a Side of Fruit & Cheese

1 Slice Whole Grain Bread (low carb.)	3	Carb.	11g
2 Tbsp. Peanut Butter	1	Protein/Fat	8g/16g
1 tsp. Jelly (low carb.)	3	Carb.	3g
1 Apple, small (or 1 serving any choice of fruit)	3	Carb.	15g
1 oz. Cheese (reduced fat)	1	Protein/Fat	7g/5g

Dinner

3 oz. Steamed Shrimp (approx. 12-16 medium-large)	1	Protein	21g
1 Cup Mixed Salad Greens	3	Carb.	5g
½ Cup Baked Potato Fries	3	Carb.	15g

Day Two

Breakfast

1 English Muffin (low-carb.)	3	Carb.	24g
(top each half with:)			
1 Poached or Fried Egg (2 eggs, total)	3	Protein	14g
1 Slice Canadian Bacon (2 slices, total)	3	Protein	14g

Lunch
Shrimp Cocktail (use leftover shrimp)

12-16 medium-large shrimp, chilled	3	Protein	21g
¼ Cup Cocktail Sauce	2	Carb.	12g
1 Cup Mixed Salad Greens	2	Carb.	5g
1-2 Tbsp Salad Dressing (any variety	--	Fat	5-10g

Dinner
Beef, Pepper and Mushroom Kabobs

(on each kabob alternate:)			
3 oz. boneless top sirloin steak (4 X 1" squares)	1	Protein	21g
4 Large mushrooms	2	Carb	3g
Red or Yellow Bell Pepper (4 X 1" pieces)	2	Carb	3g
(Note: brush each kabob with a little olive oil and lemon juice)			
½ Baked Potato, Small-Medium (serve on side)	3	Carb.	15g

Day Three

Breakfast	Plate Section #	Food Source	Grams
½ Whole Grain Bagel	3	Carb.	15g
(top Bagel with:)			
2 Scrambled Eggs (or ½ Cup Egg Substitute)		Protein	14g
1 oz. Cheese (any variety)	1	Protein	7g

Lunch

½ Turkey and Cheese Sandwich			
1 Slice Whole Grain Bread	3	Carb.	15g
3 oz. Turkey	1	Protein	21g
1 oz. Cheese	1	Protein	7g
½ Apple, small	3	Carb.	8g

Dinner

3 oz. Grilled Tuna	1	Protein	21g
1 Cup Steamed Broccoli	2	Carb.	10g
1/3 Cup Brown Rice	3	Carb.	15g

Day Four

Breakfast

2 Slices Whole Grain Toast (low carb.)	3	Carb.	22g
2 oz. Cheese (any variety; melt on top of toast)	1	Protein	14g
1 Low-Carb Yogurt	1 & 3	Protein/Carb.	7g/8g

Lunch

Chinese Chicken & Broccoli			
3 oz. chicken	1	Protein	21g
1 Cup Broccoli	2	Carb.	10g
1/3 Cup Steamed Rice	3	Carb.	15g

Dinner

Crock-pot Roast Beef, Carrots and Potatoes			
3 oz. Roast Beef	1	Protein	21g
1 Cup Stewed Carrots	2	Carb.	10g
½ Cup Stewed Potatoes	3	Carb.	15g

Day Five

Breakfast	Plate Section #	Food Source	Grams
1 Waffle (4 ½ " square)	3	Carb.	15g
½ Cup Blueberries	3	Carb.	10g
Splenda or other sugar substitute			
Scrambled Eggs (1 whole egg + ½ Cup Egg Substitute) 1		Protein	21g

Lunch
Open-Face Cheeseburger

	Plate Section #	Food Source	Grams
½ Hamburger Bun	3	Carb.	15g
3 oz. Hamburger Patty	1	Protein	21g
1 oz. Cheese	1	Protein	7g
Ketchup, Mustard and/or Mayonnaise to taste			

Dinner

	Plate Section #	Food Source	Grams
3 oz. Grilled Salmon	1	Protein	21g
1 Cup Mixed Salad Greens	2	Carb.	5g
½ Cup Boiled Red Potatoes	3	Carb.	15g
1-2 Tbsp. Salad Dressing	--	Fat	5-15g

Day Six

Breakfast

	Plate Section #	Food Source	Grams
Cantaloupe, 1/3 of a small melon	3	Carb.	15g
½ Cup Scrambled Egg Substitute	1	Protein	12g
3 Slices Bacon	1	Protein	7g

Lunch
Open-Face Tuna Melt

	Plate Section #	Food Source	Grams
1 Slice Whole Grain Toast (low carb.)	3	Carb.	11g
3 oz. Water-Packed Tuna	1	Protein	21g
1-2 Tbsp. Mayonnaise (low-fat)	--	Fat	5-10g
1 oz. Cheese (any variety	1	Protein	7g

Dinner

	Plate Section #	Food Source	Grams
Rio Grande Pot Roast (see Recipe)	1 & 2	Pro/Carb	28g/11g
1 Cup Steamed Green Beans			

Day Seven

Breakfast	Plate Section #	Food Source	Grams
Ham, Cheese and Bell Pepper Omelette			
½ Cup Egg Substitute	1	Protein	12g
1 oz. Cheese (any variety)	1	Protein	7g
1 oz. diced ham	1	Protein	7g
¼ Cup Steamed Red or Yellow Pepper	2	Carb.	3g
1 Slice Whole Grain Toast (low carb.)	3	Carb.	11g
½ Cup Strawberries (whole)	3	Carb.	7g

Lunch

	Plate Section #	Food Source	Grams
Roast Beef Sandwich			
3 oz. Leftover Roast Beef	1	Protein	21g
1 Tbsp. Mayonnaise (reduced fat)	--	Fat	5g
2 Leafs of Lettuce	2	Carb.	1g
2 Slices of Tomato	2	Carb.	2g
2 Slices Whole Grain Bread (low carb.)	3	Carb.	22g

Dinner

	Plate Section #	Food Source	Grams
Pasta Marinara with Grilled Chicken			
½ Cup Pasta (any variety)	3	Carb.	15g
½ Cup Marinara Sauce	2	Carb.	10g
3 oz. Grilled Chicken	1	Protein	21g

Recipes

Week Three

Rio Grande Pot Roast: Serves 4
¾ Cup Salsa
½ Cup Beer or Water
3 oz. tomato paste
1/2 packet taco seasoning (.75 oz., low sodium)
1.5 pound boneless round beef roast
¼ tsp. salt
¼ tsp. pepper
1 Tbsp. peanut butter
3 Tbsp. fresh cilantro (chopped)

Place salsa, beer/water, tomato paste and taco seasoning in a slow cooker. Stir to mix. Rub beef with salt and pepper. Add beef to cooker and spoon sauce mixture over meat. Cover and cook on low for 8-10 hours. Remove meat to a cutting board. Stir peanut butter and cilantro into sauce. Serve meat with sauce.

Nutrition At A Glance: Per Serving
Protein: 28 grams
Carbohydrate: 11 grams
Fat: 20 grams

Week Four

Day One

	Plate Section #	Food Source	Grams
Breakfast			
1 English Muffin (low carb)	3	Carb.	14g
2 Tbsp. Peanut Butter	1	Protein/Fat	8g/16g
1 Roll-Up (1 oz. Deli Meat + 1 oz. Cheese)	1	Protein/Fat	14g/5g

Lunch			
Grilled Chicken Sandwich (use left-over chicken)			
2 Slices Whole Grain Bread (low carb.)	3	Carb.	22g
3 oz. Chicken Breast	1	Protein	21g
1 oz. Cheese (optional)	1	Protein/Fat	21g/5g
Lettuce and Tomato	2	Carb.	3g
Mustard, Mayonnaise, Pepper (to taste)	--	--	--

Dinner			
Roasted Lemon-Pepper Pork Loin (see Recipe)	1	Protein	21-28g
Fresh Roasted Corn on the Cob (see Recipe)	3	Carb.	17g
Saute'ed Collard Greens (see Recipe)	2	Carb.	7g

Day Two

Breakfast			
¾ Cup Kashi Go Lean Crunch Cereal	1 & 3	Protein/Carb	9g/22g
½ Cup Skim or 1% Milk	1 & 3	Protein/Carb	4g/6g
1-2 Eggs (any variety)	1	Protein	7-14g

Lunch			
Lunch "On-the-go!"			
1 LUNA bar (any flavor)	1 & 2	Pro/Carb/Fat	10g/26g/4g
2 x 1 oz. Mozzarella String Cheese Sticks	1	Protein	14g

Dinner			
Herb Crusted Beef Tenderloin (see Recipe)	1	Protein	21-28g
Creamed Spinach, 1 serving (see Recipe)	2	Carb.	5g
Rosemary Roasted Potatoes, 1 serving (see Recipe)	3	Carb.	21g

Day Three

Breakfast	Plate Section #	Food Source	Grams
½ Cup Pears (or 1 Serving of any Fruit)	3	Carb.	15g
¾ Cup 1% Cottage Cheese	1	Protein	21g
12 Almonds	--	Fat	10g

Lunch			
1/2 Cup Hummus	1 & 3	Protein/Carb	7g/15g
½ of a 6" Pita	3	Carb.	15g
2 Slices Deli Meat (any variety)	1	Protein	14g

Dinner			
Saute'ed Blackened Scallops (see Recipe)	1	Protein	21-28g
Angel Hair Pasta with Lemon and Veggies	2	Carb.	24g

Day Four

Breakfast			
½ Grapefruit, large	3	Carb.	15g
1 Slice whole grain toast	3	Carb.	11g
1 oz. cheese (on toast or in eggs)	1	Protein/Fat	7g/5g
½ Cup Egg Substitute	1	Protein	12g

Lunch			
1 Cup Celery Sticks	2	Carb.	5g
2 Tbsp. Peanut Butter	1	Protein/Fat	8g/16g
2-3 Slices Deli Meat (any variety)	1	Protein	14-21g
1 Slice Whole Grain Bread	3	Carb.	11-20g

Dinner			
Shrimp Scampi with Broccoli and Red Peppers	1 & 2	Pro/Carb	28g/5g
1/3 to ½ Cup Brown or White Rice	3	Carb.	15-20g

Day Five

Breakfast	Plate Section #	Food Source	Grams
Sunny-Side Up English Muffin with Fruit			
½ English Muffin (or 1 whole low carb muffin)	3	Carb.	15g
1 Whole Egg	1	Protein	7g
1.5 oz. Cheese (any variety)	1	Protein	10g
2 oz. Canadian Bacon	1	Protein	6g
½ Cup Blueberries (or 2/3 any fruit serving)	3	Carb.	10g

Lunch

¾ Cup Low-Fat Cottage Cheese	1	Protein	21g
10 Crackers (20 grams of Carbohydrate)	3	Carb.	20g
12 Grapes	3	Carb.	10g

Dinner

Turkey Curry Meatballs	1	Protein	21-28g
¾ Cup Pasta	3	Carb.	25g

Day Six

Breakfast

2 Slices Whole Grain Toast (low carb.)	3	Carb.	22g
2 oz. Cheese (any variety; melt on top of toast)	1	Protein	14g
1 Light Yogurt ≤ 10g carbohydrate	1 & 3	Protein/Carb.	7g/8g

Lunch

Chef's Salad

1 Cup Mixed Salad Greens	2	Carb.	5g
1 boiled egg	1	Protein/Fat	7g/5g
1 oz. Cheese (any variety)	1	Protein/Fat	7g/5g
1-2 oz. of sliced chicken	1	Protein	7-14g
1-2 Tbsp. Salad Dressing (any variety)	--	Fat	5-10g
1 Slice Whole grain bread or crackers	3	Carb.	15g

Dinner

Jerk Ribs (see Recipe)	1	Protein	21-28g
1 Cup Green Beans	2	Carb	10g
½ Mashed Potatoes	3	Carb.	15g

Day Seven

Breakfast	Plate Section #	Food Source	Grams
2/3 Cup Shredded Wheat & Bran Cereal	3	Carb/Protein	24g/7g
½ Cup Skim or 1% Milk	3	Carb. Protein	6g/ 4g
2 Scrambled Eggs	1	Protein/Fat	14g/10g

Lunch
Open-Faced Tuna Melt with a Side of Fruit

1 Slice Whole Grain Toast	3	Carb.	11 g
3 oz. Tuna (water-packed)	1	Protein	21 g
1 oz. Swiss Cheese	1	Protein/Fat	6 g/ 5g
2 Tbsp. Light Mayonnaise + relish to taste	--	Fat	5-10 g
1 Small Apple (or 1 Serving of any Fruit)	3	Carb.	15 g

Dinner

Citrus Marinated Shrimp (see Recipe)	1	Protein	21-28g
1 Cup Ceasar Salad	2	Carb	5g
1 small Baked Potato	3	Carb.	20g

Recipes

Week Four

Note: *The Recipes in this section have been generously contributed by David Fouts, Bariatric Chef and author of* Culinary Classics *and* Bari-Bites. *David underwent laproscopic surgery in January of 2002 with a pre-operative weight of over 360 pounds. To hear his success story and learn more about his cook books written specifically for post-gastric-bypass patients, visit his web site at:* www.baribites.com.

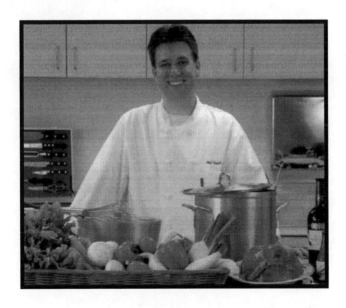

Roasted Lemon Pepper Pork Loin

Pork loin in a lemon marinade and roasted to perfection.

Servings: 8 ℰ Prep. Time: 15 min. ℰ Start to Finish: 2 hrs.

2 pounds pork loin
1 cup fresh lemon juice
2 tablespoons cracked black pepper
1 tablespoon fresh garlic, minced
1 teaspoon thyme
1 medium onion, chopped
2 tablespoons olive oil

~ Using a fork, poke holes throughout the pork loin.
~ Next, place pork loin in a large resealable bag and add remaining ingredients.
~ Let marinate for at least 4 hours, but overnight is best.
~ Place pork loin in a shallow roasting pan and pour 1 cup of marinade over pork loin.
~ Roast in oven at 350° F until roast reaches 155° F.
~ Approximate time is 1 1/2 hours.
~ Let roast stand for 15 minutes out of oven to give the juices in the roast a chance to settle.
~ Serve.
~ Yield: 4 oz.

NOTES: This is great substituted with chicken or shrimp.

Herb Crusted Beef Tenderloin

Whole beef tenderloin roasted with fresh herbs.

Servings: 12 ❦ Prep. Time: 15 min. ❦ Start to Finish: 1 hr. 30 min.

1 whole beef tenderloin, trimmed
3 tablespoons dried thyme
3 tablespoons dried basil
3 tablespoons dried oregano
3 tablespoons granulated garlic
1/4 cup olive oil
2 tablespoons salt
2 tablespoons cracked black pepper

~ Preheat oven to 375° F.
~ Next, place all ingredients, except beef, into a large mixing bowl and blend well.
~ Spread herb mix over beef tenderloin.
~ Roast on 375° F until internal temperature is 345° F (medium).
~ Yield: 6 oz.

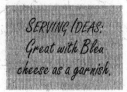

SERVING IDEAS:
Great with Bleu cheese as a garnish.

Creamed Spinach

Spinach creamed with cream cheese.

Servings: 4 ⚹ Prep. Time: 10 min. ⚹ Start to Finish: 45 min.

1 pound fresh spinach, stems removed
3 ounces cream cheese, softened
1 tablespoon melted butter
1/8 teaspoon ground nutmeg
1 tablespoon Parmesan cheeses

~ Steam spinach until leaves are tender; drain well.
~ Combine cream cheese, butter and nutmeg and stir well.
~ Stir in spinach, spoon into lightly greased 1-quart casserole pan, sprinkle with Parmesan cheese.
~ Cover and bake at 350° F for 20 minutes.
~ Yield: 4 oz.

NOTES: You can substitute with collard or mustard greens.

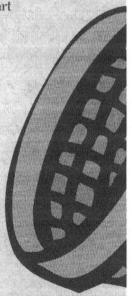

SERVING IDEAS:
To spice up your creamed spinach add a diced jalapeño. Goes great with a grilled ribeye steak.

Rosemary Roasted Potatoes

Red potatoes roasted with rosemary.

Servings: 8 ❦ Prep. Time: 15 min. ❦ Start to Finish: 1 hr.

4 pounds red potatoes, cut in 2" pieces
1/4 cup olive oil
3 tablespoons fresh rosemary, chopped fine
1 tablespoon fresh thyme, chopped fine
2 tablespoons fresh garlic, minced
2 teaspoons paprika
Salt and pepper, to taste

~ Place all ingredients in a large mixing
  bowl and mix well.
~ Next, place mixed potatoes
  into a large roasting pan.
~ Preheat oven to 375° F.
~ Place potatoes in oven and roast uncovered
  for 45 minutes or until tender, turning every
  15 minutes to brown evenly on all sides.
~ Yield: 4 oz.

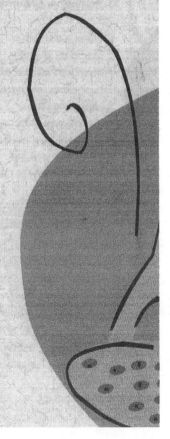

SERVING IDEAS:
Great with herbed
roasted tenderloin.

Sautéed Blackened Scallops

Spicy scallops sautéed in butter.

Servings: 4 ✿ Prep. Time: 5 min. ✿ Start to Finish: 30 min.

1 pound scallops
1/2 stick butter

<u>Blackening Spices</u>
1 teaspoon salt
3/4 teaspoon black pepper
1/2 teaspoon white pepper
3/4 teaspoon dry mustard
1 tablespoon garlic powder
1/2 teaspoon dried thyme
2 teaspoon paprika

SERVING IDEAS: Garnish with a lemon wedge.

- Mix blackening spices together.
- Dredge scallops in blackening spices.
- In skillet, sauté scallops on high heat for 6 to 8 minutes.
- Yield: 4 oz.

NOTES: Add less pepper if you don't want seasoning so hot.

Angel Hair Pasta with Lemon and Veggies

Pasta with veggies, lemon and Parmesan cheese.

Servings: 8 ❦ Prep. Time: 15 min. ❦ Start to Finish: 20 min.

1 medium zucchini, cubed
1 medium tomato, chopped
1 tablespoon butter
1/2 cup mushrooms, sliced
1/2 cup onions, chopped
1/2 cup red bell pepper, chopped
2 cups angel hair pasta, cooked
6 large basil leaves, chopped
1/4 cup fresh lemon juice
1/2 cup Parmesan cheese
Salt and pepper, to taste

> *SERVING IDEAS:*
> *Garnish with chopped scallions and grilled chicken or shrimp.*

~ In a large sauté pan over high heat add butter.
~ Once butter has melted, add all the vegetables.
~ Sauté for 7 to 8 minutes.
~ Next add cooked pasta, lemon juice, basil, Parmesan cheese, salt and pepper; sauté for 5 minutes.
~ Yield: 4 oz.

NOTES: This is also great served cold.

Shrimp Scampi with Broccoli and Red Peppers

Broccoli and red bell pepper sautéed with shrimp.

Servings: 8 ❀ Prep. Time: 10 min. ❀ Start to Finish: 15 min.

1 1/2 pounds shrimp, peeled
2 tablespoons olive oil
2 cloves fresh garlic, peeled and chopped
1 pinch salt and pepper
1 teaspoon paprika
1 cup broccoli florets
1 large red bell pepper, chopped

- In a large sauté pan, heat olive oil over medium-high heat.
- Next, add broccoli, red bell pepper, garlic, and sauté for 3 to 5 minutes.
- Add shrimp and sauté for 3 to 5 additional minutes.
- Shrimp is done when color becomes creamy white.
- Sprinkle with paprika, parsley, salt and pepper.
- Serve.
- Yield: 4 oz.

SERVING IDEAS:
Serve with a side of steamed rice.
Chicken can also be used.

Per Serving : 257 Calories; 10g Fat (35.3% calories from fat); 35g Protein; 5g Carbohydrate; 1g Dietary Fiber; 259mg Cholesterol; 280mg Sodium. Exchanges: 0 Grain (Starch); 5 Lean Meat; 1/2 Vegetable; 1 1/2 Fat.

Turkey Curry Meatballs

Spicy turkey meatballs with Romano cheese.

Servings: 4 ❦ Prep. Time: 15 min. ❦ Start to Finish: 45 min.

1 pound ground turkey
1 teaspoon curry powder
1 tablespoon hot sauce
1/2 cup Romano cheese
1 teaspoon fresh garlic, minced
1 tablespoon onion powder
1 teaspoon chili powder
1 large egg
Salt and pepper, to taste

~ In a large mixing bowl combine all ingredients and mix well.
~ Next roll meatball mixture into 2" round balls.
~ Place meatballs in a shallow pan and bake at 350° F for 30 minutes.
~ Serve.
~ Yield: 4 oz.

NOTES : Wet your hands first when rolling your meatballs; this keeps the meat from sticking to your hands.

SERVING IDEAS:
These meatballs can be made ahead of time and baked later. Great for parties.

Jerk Ribs

Spicy pork ribs.

Servings: 4 ❦ Prep. Time: 10 min. ❦ Start to Finish: 1 hr. 30 min.

2 pounds pork back ribs
2 tablespoons dried minced onion
1 tablespoon onion powder
4 teaspoons ground thyme
2 teaspoons salt
2 teaspoons ground allspice
1/2 teaspoon ground nutmeg
1/2 teaspoon ground cinnamon
1 tablespoon sugar substitute
2 teaspoons black pepper
1 teaspoon cayenne pepper

– In a small jar with tight-fitting lid, shake together
   all dry ingredients until well-blended.
– Rub dry mixture onto all surfaces of ribs.
– Grill ribs in covered grill, turning occasionally,
   until ribs are very tender, about 1 1/2 hours.
– Yield: 4 oz.

NOTES: Or roast ribs on rack in shallow pan in 350° F oven for 1 1/2 hours.

SERVING IDEAS:
Great with a wedge of sharp Cheddar cheese.

Marinated Grilled Shrimp

Citrus-marinated jumbo shrimp on skewers.

Servings: 4 ☙ Prep. Time: 20 min. ☙ Start to Finish: 3 hrs.

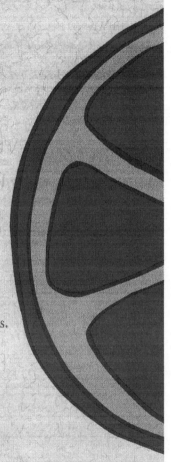

1 pound jumbo shrimp, peeled
2 cloves fresh garlic, minced
2 tablespoons olive oil
2 tablespoons hot sauce
1/4 cup fresh lemon juice
1/4 cup fresh orange juice
1/4 cup scallions, chopped fine
2 tablespoons fresh dill, chopped fine
4 skewers
Salt, to taste
Cracked black pepper, to taste

- Place 4 ounces of shrimp on a skewer.
- Next, place skewed shrimp into air-tight container and add remaining ingredients.
- Let marinate at least 2 hours.
- Place shrimp on grill over medium coals and cook 3 minutes each side.
- Shrimp may take longer to cook depending on size.
- Yield: 4 oz.

SERVING IDEAS:
Great served over a fresh Caesar salad.

Appendix G

Frozen Dinners
Already Built for You ...Using the "Plate Method"

Product	Carbohydrate	Protein
Healthy Choice		
Mushroom Roasted Beef	28g	23g
Oven-Roasted Beef	33g	22g
Grilled Turkey Breast	31g	18g
Lean Cuisine		
Spa Classics		
Chicken and Vegetables	27g	20g
Chicken Carbonara	35g	20g
Fiesta Grilled Chicken	27g	19g
Weight Watchers		
Smart Ones		
*Chicken Marsala w/ Broccoli	10g	20g
*Salisbury Steak	12g	20g
Lasagne Florentine	35g	15g *(add 1 oz. of meat or 7 grams of protein)*

* To ensure adequate calories, include a side of vegetables, bread, fruit or other carbohydrate to increase your total carbohydrate to 30 grams per meal.

Meal Replacement Bars
Appropriate for Use in Moderation
When Eating "On-the-Go!"

Product	Carb.	Protein	Add this Amount of Protein to meet Minimum Goal of 21 grams/meal
Atkins	22g	18g	<1 Serving (3g)
Balance	21g	16g	1 Serving (7g
Body for Life	21g	15g	1 Serving (7g)
CLIF (2/3 of a bar)	30g	7g	2 Servings (14g)
CLIF Builder's	30g	20g	---
EAS AdvantEdge	23g	21g	---
Kashi-Go-Lean	30g	9g	2 Servings (14g)
Luna	24g	10g	1.5 Servings (11g)
Pure Protein	19g	19g	---
South Beach	26g	19g	---
Zone	23g	16g	1 Serving (7g)

Note: *The nutritional content may vary within each product brand based on the flavor you choose.*

• To meet your minimum protein goal of 21 grams per meal, complement your meal replacement bar with additional protein servings as noted above.
Example 1: Eat 1 oz. of cheese with your Balance bar.
Example 2: Eat 2 slices of deli meat with your Kashi bar.

• To ensure adequate calories add additional carbohydrate up to 30 grams per meal, as needed.
Example 1: Eat 8-10 grapes with your Zone bar.
Example 2: Eat 2/3 banana with your Pure Protein bar.

Appendix H

Spinach Salad Recipe

Dressing
¼ Cup Scallions, thinly sliced
¼ Cup Soy Sauce
¼ Cup Rice Vinegar
2 Tbsp. Water
2 Cloves Garlic, minced
2 tsp. toasted Sesame Seeds
2 tsp. toasted Sesame Oil
1 tsp. Chili Paste

Salad
2 tsp. toasted Sesame Oil
6 Scallions, chopped into one inch pieces
¾ pound Shiitake Mushroom caps, sliced
3 Cups Corn
3 Cups Bean Sprouts
2 Red Bell Peppers, sliced thinly
18 Cups rinsed Spinach Leaves
Cooking Spray

Top With
4 oz. of salmon, tuna or chicken, grilled

Preheat broiler. Whisk together dressing ingredients in a small bowl and set aside. Heat oil in a large non-stick skillet over medium-high heat. Add scallions and mushrooms. Saute' for 6 minutes. Stir in corn, cover and set aside. Prepare salmon, tuna or chicken. Divide spinach, bean sprouts and peppers among six plates. Top with an equal portion of warm mushroom mixture, 4 oz. of meat and dressing. Serve immediately and enjoy!

Appendix I

Sample Aerobic Programs

Getting Started: Moderate Intensity Cardio, Maintaining a Consistent Intensity Level

Strategy: You will maintain a steady, moderate pace for the entire workout. This would be equivalent to an RPE between 5 and 6 or the low to mid-point of your THR range (65-75% MHR.)

Benefit: Exercising aerobically for 30-60 minutes at a steady, moderate pace helps you build a base of cardiovascular fitness and helps you burn more calories each day you are active.

"Hold It Steady"
Sample Steady State Beginner Treadmill Workout:

Time	Focus	RPE
5-8 min.	Warm-up with an easy walking pace.	3
15-30 min.	Increase your walking speed and/or the treadmill incline until you reach a moderate effort level (the middle to lower end of your THR.)	5-6
5 min.	Cool-down	3

Note: Warm-up and cool-down with 5 minutes or so of a low intensity level of whatever aerobic activity you are doing that day (e.g. slow walking on the treadmill, slow-deliberate stair climbing, easy cycling, or easy lap-swimming.) Think of your warm-up as a time to increase blood flow and prepare your muscles for the workout ahead. Likewise, your cool-down is a time to clear lactic acid and other waste products from the muscles and prepare them for stretching.

Six-Week Program to Build Cardio Fitness
Walk at a moderate pace with an RPE of 5-6.

Week	W/U	Walk	C/D	Total	# of Days
1	5-8 min.	15 min.	5 min.	25-28 min.	2-3
2	5-8 min.	20 min.	5 min.	30-33 min.	2-3
3	5-8 min.	20 min.	5 min.	30-33 min.	3
4	5-8 min.	25 min.	5 min.	35-38 min.	3-4
5	5-8 min.	30 min.	5 min.	40-43 min.	3-5
6	5-8 min.	35 min.	5 min.	45-48 min.	3-5

Interval Training – Taking It Up a Notch!

Strategy: You will vary the intensity of your workout by alternating between moderate and high intensity intervals with rest periods in between.

Benefit: Interval training will teach your cardiovascular system to tolerate higher exercise intensities and improve your overall fitness level. Interval training burns more calories than steady-state cardio and even leaves your metabolism elevated for a period of time following the workout. Thus interval training burns more calories both during and after your workout session.

Sample Interval Workout on a Treadmill

Intermediate Level: 30-33 minutes
Estimated Calorie burn: 250-350

Time	Focus	RPE
5-8 min.	Warm-up with an easy walking pace.	3
5 min.	Slightly increase your pace or incline.	5
1 min.	Increase your intensity.	7-8
2 min.	Resume moderate intensity and recover	5
1 min.	Increase your intensity.	7-8
2 min.	Resume moderate intensity and recover	5
1 min.	Increase your intensity.	7-8
2 min.	Resume moderate intensity and recover	5
1 min.	Increase your intensity.	7-8
2 min.	Resume moderate intensity and recover	5
1 min.	Increase your intensity.	7-8
2 min.	Resume moderate intensity and recover	5
5 min.	Cool-down with an easy walking pace.	2-3
5 min.	Finish with stretches to target your quadriceps, hamstrings, calves and lower back.	

Note: to increase the intensity of your interval workout, decrease your rest time between intervals and/or increase the number of intervals performed. To decrease workout intensity, increase rest time between intervals and/or decrease the number of intervals performed.

Sample Interval Workout on a Stair Climber
Intermediate Level: 25-28 minutes
Estimated Calorie burn: 300-400

Time	Focus	RPE
5-8 minutes	Climb with an easy pace	3
3 minutes	Slightly increase your climbing pace.	5
20 seconds	Increase your intensity to upper end of THR.	7-8
1 minute	Resume moderate intensity and recover.	5
20 seconds	Increase your intensity to upper end of THR.	7-8
1 minute	Resume moderate intensity and recover.	5
20 seconds	Increase your intensity to upper end of THR.	7-8
1 minute	Resume moderate intensity and recover.	5
20 seconds	Increase your intensity to upper end of THR.	7-8
1 minute	Resume moderate intensity and recover.	5
20 seconds	Increase your intensity to upper end of THR.	7-8
1 minute	Resume moderate intensity and recover.	5
20 seconds	Increase your intensity to upper end of THR.	7-8
5 minutes	Resume moderate intensity and recover.	5
5 minutes	Cool-down	2-3
5 minutes	Finish with stretches to target your quadriceps, hamstrings, calves and lower back.	

(Continue Next Page)

Sample Six-Week Program Introducing Interval Training

Week	Steady State	Intervals	Total Cardio Days
1	2-3	1	3-4
2	2-3	1-2	3-5
3-4	2-3	2	4-5
5-6	3	2	5

Note: This program can be used with any aerobic activity. Choose an aerobic activity you have a good base of fitness with and step-it-up a notch.

Eight-Week Program to Increase Running Endurance

Goal: "I want to be able to run three miles without stopping."

Week	Walk	Run	Repeat	Walk	Total
1	5 min.	2 min.	2X	5 min.	26 min.
2	5 min.	4 min.	2X	5 min.	32 min.
3	4 min.	6 min.	2X	5 min.	35 min.
4	3 min.	8 min.	2X	5 min.	38 min.
5	2 min.	10 min.	2X	5 min.	41 min.
6	1 min.	12 min.	2X	5 min.	44 min.
7	1 min.	14 min.	1X	5 min.	35 min.
8	1 min.	30 min.	0	5 min.	36 min.

Note: Do each week's routine three times, with at least one day of rest in between. By gradually increasing your running time, you will be able to jog 30 consecutive minutes in approximately two months.

Appendix J

Sample Resistance Training Programs

In this section you will find programs to target the **front-upper body** (chest, triceps and anterior deltoids), **back-upper body** (lats, rhomboids, biceps and medial and posterior deltoids), **lower body** (quadriceps, hamstrings and glutes), **total body** (all of the muscle groups mentioned above) and the **abdominals**.

The beginner and intermediate programs are six-week progressive programs that will improve your strength and muscle tone without the risk of injury from over-doing it. I've also included advanced programs for the more experienced exerciser and some non-gym "break-out" workouts for use when traveling or when you just can't make it to the gym.

There is no one correct way to sequence your resistance exercises. The most important thing is to start with a program appropriate for your current fitness level and gradually increase your intensity (and variety) to avoid fitness plateaus. If you prefer to create your own program, you may want to consider using some of the sample program templates listed at the end of this section.

Finally, we have included pictures to visually demonstrate some of the core exercises included in these resistance programs. Visit our web-site for more pictures and written guidelines for executing many of the exercises included in Appendix J: www.theroadtowlssuccess.com

Muscles of the Front-Body

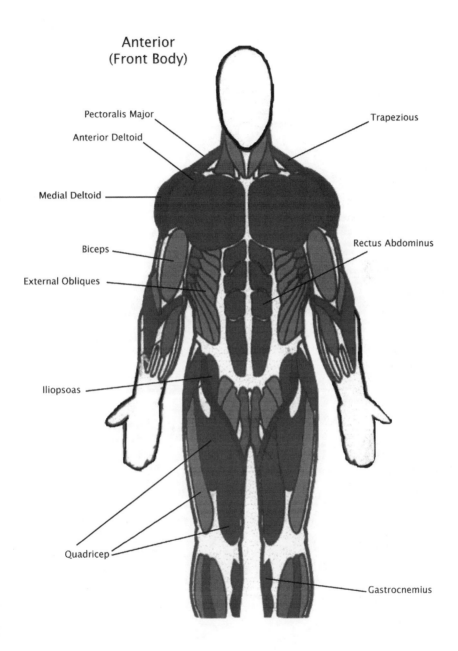

Anterior
(Front Body)

Pectoralis Major

Anterior Deltoid

Trapezious

Medial Deltoid

Biceps

Rectus Abdominus

External Obliques

Iliopsoas

Quadricep

Gastrocnemius

Muscles of the Back-Body

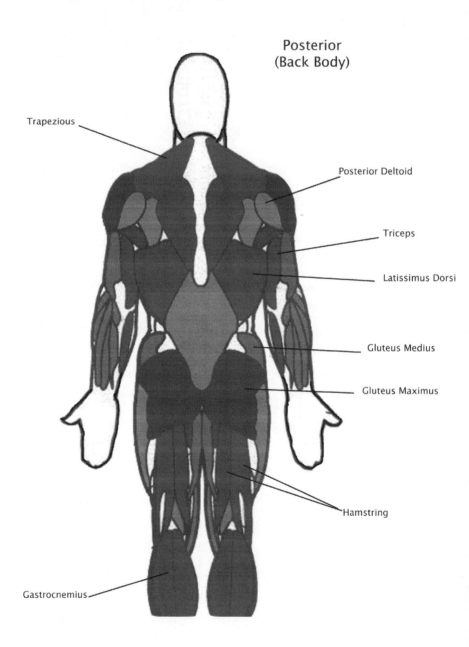

Posterior
(Back Body)

Trapezious

Posterior Deltoid

Triceps

Latissimus Dorsi

Gluteus Medius

Gluteus Maximus

Hamstring

Gastrocnemius

Total Body: Beginner Workouts

This is a progressive six-week program using moderate weight to build strength and muscle tone in all the major muscle groups of the body. Targeting large muscle groups is an efficient way to train because it maximizes the number of calories you burn both during and after your workout session, with less time spent in the gym. Perform two total body exercises or alternate with your split routines.

Week	Exercise	Sets	Reps
Do one set of each exercise in a series back to back; rest 45 to 90 seconds and then repeat or ove on to the second series:			
1 and 2	**Series One**		
	Ball Squat on Wall	2	12-15
	Modified Push-Up	2	12-15
	Assisted Pull-Up	2	12-15
3 and 4	**Series One**		
	Ball Squat on Wall	1-2	12-15
	Modified Push-Up	1-2	12-15
	Assisted Pull-Up	1-2	12-15
	Series Two		
	Stationary Lunges	2	10-12
	Seated Chest Press	2	10-12
	Stack Row	2	10-12
5 and 6	**Series One**		
	Ball Squat on Wall	2	12-15
	Ball Push-Up on Thigh	2	12-15
	Assisted Pull-Up	2	12-15
	Series Two		
	Leg Press	2-3	10-12
	Flat Bench Press	2-3	10-12
	Seated Cable Row	2-3	10-12

Note: Choose a weight heavy enough to fatigue the targeted muscles by the last 2-3 reps; rest 45 to 60 seconds between sets.

Total Body: Intermediate Workouts

This is a six-week program using moderate weight with progressively increasing intensity. Do the exercises listed twice a week.

Week	Exercise	Sets	Reps
1 and 2	*Do one set of each exercise in a series back to back; rest 45 to 90 seconds and then repeat:*		
	Ball Squat on Wall	2-3	10-12
	Romanian Dead Lift	2-3	10-12
	Seated Chest Press	2-3	10-12
	Stack Row	2-3	10-12
3 and 4	**Super-Set each pair of exercises**:**		
	Smith Machine Squat	2-3	12-15
	Ball Squat on Wall	2-3	12-15
	Flat Bench Press	2-3	10-12
	Ball Push up (on thigh or shin)	2-3	to fatigue
	Assisted Pull-Up	2-3	10-12
	Lat Pull-Down	2-3	10-12
5 and 6	**Super-Set each pair of exercises:**		
	Unilateral Walking Lunges	3	10-15
	Ball Squat on Wall	3	10-15
	Incline Barbell Press	3	10-12
	Flat Bench Dumbbell Fly	3	10-12
	Seated Cable Row	3	10-12
	Bent-Over Dumbbell Fly	3	10-12

Note: Choose a weight heavy enough to fatigue the targeted muscles by the last 2-3 reps; rest 45 to 60 seconds between sets.

** **A Super-Set** consists of two different exercises targeting the same muscle groups (or opposing muscle groups) performed back-to-back without rest

Back-Upper Body: Beginner Workouts

This is a progressive six-week program using moderate weight to build strength and muscle tone in the back-upper body muscles including: the lats, rhomboids, biceps and medial and posterior deltoids. Do the exercises listed twice a week.

Week	Exercise	Sets	Reps
1 and 2	Lat Pull-Down	1-2	12-15
	Stack Row	1-2	12-15
3 and 4	Assisted Pull-Up	2	12-15
	Seated Cable Row	2	10-12
5 and 6	Warm-Up: Assisted Pull-Up	1	12-15
	Lat Pull-Down	2	10-12
	Seated Cable Row	2	10-12
	Stack Row	2	10-12

Note: Choose a weight heavy enough to fatigue the targeted muscles by the last two or three repetitions of each set; rest 45 to 60 seconds between sets.

As the exercises get noticeably easier and you experience less delayed onset muscle soreness, you should add a little **over-load** to avoid a fitness plateau. After six consecutive weeks on this program, or when you are ready for a little more challenge, transition to the intermediate workouts.

Back-Upper Body: Intermediate Workouts

This is a six-week program using moderate weight with progressively increasing intensity. Do the exercises listed twice a week.

Week	Exercise	Sets	Reps
1 and 2	Assisted Pull-Up	2-3	12-15
	Seated Cable Row	2	10-12
	Bent-Over Dumbbell Flies	2	10-12
3 and 4	Warm-Up: Assisted Pull-Up	2	12-15
	Narrow-Grip Pull-Down	2	10-12
	One-Arm Stack Row	2	10-12
	Bent-Over Barbell Row	2	10-12
5 and 6	*Alternate the following workouts*:		
	Workout One		
	Warm-Up: Assisted Pull-Up	2	10-12
	Lat Pull Down	2-3	10-12
	Bent-Over Barbell Row	2-3	10-12
	Bent-Over Dumbbell Flies	2-3	10-12
	Workout Two		
	Narrow-Grip Pull-Down	2-3	10-12
	One Arm Dumbbell Row	2-3	10-12
	Seated Cable Row	2-3	10-12
	One-Arm Stack Row	2-3	10-12

Note: Choose a weight heavy enough to fatigue the targeted muscles by the last two or three repetitions of each set; rest 45 to 60 seconds between sets. After six consecutive weeks on this program, or when you need more over-load, transition to the advanced workouts.

Back-Upper Body: Advanced Workouts

Perform two work-outs a week, alternating the following programs.

Exercise	Sets	Reps
Workout One		
Assisted Pull-Up	2-3	8-12
Drop-Set Each Exercise*		
Narrow Grip Pull-Down	3	10/5
Seated Cable Row	3	10/5
Bent-Over Dumbbell Flies	3	10/5
One Arm Seated Cable Row	3	10/5
Workout Two		
Assisted Pull-Up	2-3	8-12
Bent-Over Barbell Row	3	8-12
One-Arm Dumbbell Row	3	8-12
Drop Set Each Exercise		
One-Arm Stack Row	3	10/5
Lat Pull-Down	3	10/5

Note: Choose a weight heavy enough to fatigue the targeted muscles by the last two or three repetitions of each set; rest 60 to 90 seconds between sets.

* **Drop-Set:** start the first set with enough weight to fatigue by the tenth repetition. Then, without rest, decrease the weight and complete an additional five repetitions.

Back-Upper Body: Break-Out Workouts!

Perform the following exercises to target the back, biceps and rear shoulder muscles on days when you are traveling, unable to get to the gym or just want a change of scenery.

Exercise	Sets	Reps
One-Arm Dumbbell Row	2-3	8-15
Bent-Over Dumbbell Flies	2-3	8-15
Lat Pull-Down (use resistance tubing)	2-3	8-15
Seated Row (use resistance tubing)	2-3	8-15
Bicep Curls (use resistance tubing)	2-3	8-15
Bent-Over Row* (use a dumbbell or barbell)	2-3	8-15
Pull-Up* (use a pull-up bar in a doorjamb)	2-3	5-15

Note: In place of dumbbells substitute other hand held, weighted objects such as soup cans, bags filled with sand, water-filled milk cartons or medicine balls.

Note: Exercises marked with an asterisk (*) are advanced and should not be performed by beginners.

Front-Upper Body: Beginner Workouts

This is a progressive six-week program using moderate weight to build strength and muscle tone in the front-upper body muscles including: the chest, triceps and anterior deltoids. Do the exercises listed twice a week.

Week	Exercise	Sets	Reps
1 and 2	Modified Push-Up	2	10-15
	Seated Chest-Press	2	10-12
3 and 4	Modified Push-Up	2	10-15
	Seated Chest-Press	2-3	10-12
	Incline Dumbbell Press	2	10-12
5 and 6	Ball Push-ups on Thighs	2	12-15
	Barbell Bench Press	2	10-12
	Flat Bench Dumbbell Fly	2	10-12

Note: Choose a weight heavy enough to fatigue the targeted muscles by the last two or three repetitions of each set; rest 45 to 60 seconds between sets.

As the exercises get noticeably easier and you experience less delayed onset muscle soreness, you should add a little **over-load** to avoid a fitness plateau. After six consecutive weeks on this program, or when you are ready for a little more challenge, transition to the intermediate workouts.

Front-Upper Body: Intermediate Workouts

This is a six-week program using moderate weight with progressively increasing intensity. Do the exercises listed twice a week.

Week	Exercise	Sets	Reps
1 and 2	Ball Push-Ups on Shins	2-3	12-15
	Incline Dumbbell Press	2-3	10-12
	Flat Bench Dumbbell Fly	2-3	10-12
3 and 4	Full or Ball Push-Up	2	12-15
	Pyramid Set*		
	Barbell Bench Press	1st	12-15
		2nd	10-12
		3rd	8 -10
	Super-Set**		
	Flat Bench Dumbbell Fly	2-3	10-12
	Incline Dumbbell Press	2-3	10-12
5 and 6	Super-Set		
	Barbell Bench Press	2-3	10-12
	Full or Ball Push-Up	2-3	(to fatigue)
	Super-Set		
	Incline Dumbbell Fly	2-3	10-12
	Flat Bench Cable Fly	2-3	10-12

Note: Choose a weight heavy enough to fatigue the targeted muscles by the last two or three repetitions of each set; rest 45 to 60 seconds between sets. After six consecutive weeks on this program, or when you need more over-load, transition to the advanced workouts.

* **A Pyramid** is three or more sets of an exercise using progressively heavier weights while performing fewer reps. For instance, for your first set choose a moderate weight that challenges you between twelve to fifteen reps (for maximum calorie burn) or eight to ten reps (to increase muscle size.) On your second set, increase the weight and perform ten to twelve reps or six to eight reps. On your final set, increase the weight again and perform eight to ten reps or four to six reps. You can reverse

240

the pyramid, moving from high weight and low reps to low weight and high reps, to maximize the variety and over-load of your workouts.

** **A Super-Set** consists of two different exercises targeting the same muscle groups (or opposing muscle groups) performed back-to-back without rest.

Front-Upper Body: Advanced Workouts

Perform two work-outs a week, alternating the following programs.

Exercise	Sets	Reps
Workout One		
Full Push-Up	2-3	8-12
(with hands on the floor or on a balance board)		
Pyramid Set:		
Incline Dumbbell Press	1st	12-15
	2nd	10-12
	3rd	8-10
Super-Set:		
Barbell Bench Press	3	10-12
Flat-Bench Dumbbell Fly	3	10-12
Workout Two		
Full Push-Up	2-3	12-15
(With feet slightly elevated on a step)		
Pyramid Set:		
Incline Bench Press	1st	12-15
	2nd	10-12
	3rd	8-10
Super-Set:		
Flat Bench Dumbbell Fly	3	10-12
Standing Cable Fly	3	10-12

Note: Choose a weight heavy enough to fatigue the targeted muscles by the last two or three repetitions of each set; rest 60 to 90 seconds between sets.

Front-Upper Body: Break-Out Workouts!

Perform the following exercises to target the chest, triceps and front shoulder muscles on days when you are traveling, unable to get to the gym or just want a change of scenery.

Exercise	Sets	Reps
Push-Up (Modified, Full, Ball or Incline)	2-3	10-15
Dumbbell Press (on a bench, ball or floor)	2-3	10-15
Dumbbell Fly (on a bench, ball or floor)	2-3	10-15
Seated Chest Press (with resistance tubing)	2-3	10-15
Seated Flies (with resistance tubing)	2-3	10-15
Tricep Dips (on the side of a bath tub or a stable piece of furniture)	2-3	10-15

Note: In place of dumbbells substitute other hand held, weighted objects such as soup cans, bags filled with sand, water-filled milk cartons or medicine balls.

Lower Body: Beginner Workouts

This is a progressive six-week program using moderate weight to build strength and muscle tone in the lower- body muscles including: the quadriceps, hamstrings and glutes. Do the exercises listed twice a week.

Week	Exercise	Sets	Reps
1 and 2	Ball Squat on Wall	2	12-15
	Prone Hamstring Curl	2	12-15
	Unilateral Stationary Lunge	2	12-15
3 and 4	Ball Squat on Wall	2	12-15
	Seated Hamstring Curl	2	12-15
	Plie' Dumbbell Squat	2	12-15
	Unilateral Walking Lunge	2	12-15
5 and 6	Alternate the following workouts:		
	Workout One		
	Ball Squat on Wall	2	12-15
	Leg Press	2	12-15
	Prone Hamstring Curl	2	12-15
	Unilateral Walking Lunge	2	12-15
	Workout Two		
	Plie' Dumbbell Squat	2	12-15
	Smith-Machine Squat	2	12-15
	Seated Hamstring Curl	2	12-15
	Unilateral Stationary Lunge	2	12-15

Note: Choose a weight heavy enough to fatigue the targeted muscles by the last two or three repetitions of each set; rest 45 to 60 seconds between sets.

As the exercises get noticeably easier and you experience less delayed onset muscle soreness, you should add a little over-load to avoid a fitness plateau. After six consecutive weeks on this program, or when you are ready for a little more challenge, transition to the intermediate workouts.

Lower Body: Intermediate Workouts

Do the exercises listed twice a week.

Week	Exercise	Sets	Reps
1 and 2	Ball Squat on Wall	2-3	12-15
	Unilateral Reverse Lunge	2-3	12-15
	Drop Set*:		
	Prone Hamstring Curl	2	10/5
	Plie' Squat	2	10/5
3 and 4	Leg Press	2-3	12-15
	Smith Machine Squat	2-3	12-15
	Unilateral Prone Ham Curl	2-3	12-15
	Drop Set:		
	Seated Hamstring Curl	2	10/5
5 and 6	Super-Set**:		
	Ball Squat on Wall	2-3	12-15
	Unilateral Walking Lunge	2-3	12-15
	Super-Set:		
	Romanian Dead Lift	2-3	12-15
	Unilateral Seated Ham Curl	2-3	12-15
	Drop-Set:		
	Leg Press	2	10/5

Note: Choose a weight heavy enough to fatigue the targeted muscles by the last two or three repetitions of each set; rest 45 to 60 seconds between sets. After six consecutive weeks on this program, or when you need more over-load, transition to the advanced workouts.

* **Drop-Set:** start the first set with enough weight to fatigue the target muscles by the tenth repetition. Then, without rest, decrease the weight and complete an additional five repetitions.

** **A Super-Set** consists of two different exercises targeting the same muscle groups (or opposing muscle groups) performed back-to-back without rest.

Lower-Body: Advanced Workouts

Perform two work-outs a week, alternating the following programs.

Exercise	Sets	Reps
Workout One		
Super-Set:		
Squat	3	12-15
Unilateral Walking Lunge	3	12-15
Step-Up with Knee Lift	3	12-15
Multiple-Drop-Set*:		
Leg Press	2-3	10/5/5
Workout Two		
One-Legged Squat	2-3	12-15
Super-Set:		
Reverse Lunge	2-3	12-15
Romanian Dead Lift	2-3	12-15
Multiple-Drop-Set:		
Prone Hamstring Curl	2-3	10/5/5

Note: Choose a weight heavy enough to fatigue the targeted muscles by the last two or three repetitions of each set; rest 60 to 90 seconds between sets.

* Multiple-Drop-Set: start the first set with enough weight to fatigue the target muscles by the tenth repetition. Without rest, decrease the weight and complete an additional five repetitions. Again, decrease the weight and complete an additional five reps.

Lower-Body: Break-Out Workouts!

Perform the following exercises to target the lower-body muscles and stimulate your metabolism on days when you are traveling, unable to get to the gym or just want a change of scenery.

Exercise	Sets	Reps
Free Standing or Ball-on-Wall Squat	2-3	12-15
Romanian Dead Lift	2-3	12-15
Plie' Squat	2-3	12-15
Unilateral Walking Lunge	2-3	12-15
Leg Extension (with tubing)	2-3	12-15
Standing Hamstring Curl (with tubing)	2-3	12-15
Super-Set:		
Unilateral Reverse Lunge	2-3	12-15
Unilateral Step-Up	2-3	12-15

Note: In place of dumbbells substitute other hand held, weighted objects such as soup cans, bags filled with sand, water-filled milk cartons or medicine balls.

Abdominals: Beginner Workouts

This is a progressive, six-week program. Do the following exercises 2 times per week; rest 45-60 seconds between all sets or super-sets. Progress to the intermediate workouts for more of a challenge.

Week	Exercise	Sets	Reps
1 and 2	Ball Rollback Crunch	2	8-15
	Cross-Body Crunch	1-2	8-15
	Indian-Style Floor Crunch	1-2	8-15
3 and 4	Ball Crunch	2	10-15
	Reverse Crunch	2	10-15
	Oblique Crunch	2	10-15
5 and 6	Super-Set** each pair of exercises:		
	Floor Crunch with a		
	Reverse Crunch	2	10-15
	Reverse Crunch	2	10-15
	Oblique Crunch	2	10-15
	Decline Oblique Twist	2	10-15

Note: Always exhale (blow out) on exertion (the lift or work phase) and inhale (breathe in) as you release the contraction (lower back down to the floor.) Focus on holding the contraction of each exercise for the entire duration of your exhale. Then, resist gravity as you inhale and slowly lower your body back down to the floor to begin your next rep.

** A Super-Set consists of two or more different exercises targeting the same muscle groups (or opposing muscle groups) performed back-to-back without rest.

Abdominals: Intermediate Workouts

This is a progressive, six-week program. Do the following exercises 2-4 times per week; rest 45-60 seconds between all sets or super-sets.

Week	Exercise	Sets	Reps
1 and 2	Super-Set**:		
	Weighted Ball Crunch	2-3	10-15
	Medicine-Ball Reverse Crunch	2-3	10-15
	Plank-to-Knee Tuck	2-3	10-15
3 and 4	Super-Set:		
	Floor Crunch with Medicine-		
	Ball Reverse Crunch	3	10-15
	Medicine-Ball Oblique Crunch	3	10-15
	Reverse Crunch	3	10-15
	Plank-to-Knee Tuck	3	(to fatigue)
5 and 6	Super-Set:		
	Weighted Ball Crunch	3	10-15
	Medicine-Ball Reverse Crunch	3	10-15
	Plank-to-Knee Oblique Tuck	3	10-15
	Pilates-100		

Note: Always exhale (blow out) on exertion (the lift or work phase) and inhale (breathe in) as you release the contraction (lower back down to the floor.) Focus on holding the contraction of each exercise for the entire duration of your exhale. Then, resist gravity as you inhale and slowly lower your body back down to the floor to begin your next rep.

** A Super-Set consists of two or more different exercises targeting the same muscle groups (or opposing muscle groups) performed back-to-back without rest.

Remember to add variety and apply the F.I.T. principle to continue making progress.

Sample Templates for Creating Your Own Resistance Training Routines

Sample Total Body Schedule:

Day 1: Total Body
Day 2: Off or Cardio Only
Day 3: Off or Cardio Only
Day 4: Total Body
Day 5: Off or Cardio Only
Day 6: Off or Cardio Only
Day 7: Off

Sample Upper/Lower-Body Schedule:

	Beginner/Intermediate	Advanced
Day 1:	Upper	Upper
Day 2:	Off or Cardio Only	Lower
Day 3:	Lower	Off or Cardio Only
Day 4:	Off or Cardio Only	Upper
Day 5:	Upper	Lower
Day 6:	Off or Cardio Only	Off or Cardio Only
Day 7:	Off or Cardio Only	Off or Cardio Only

Note: *Start the next week with the lower-body routine and follow the same schedule.*

Sample Opposing Muscle Groups Schedule:

Day 1: Front-Upper Body and Back-Upper Body
Day 2: Off or Cardio Only
Day 3: Lower Body: with a focus on Quadriceps vs. Hamstrings
Day 4: Off or Cardio Only
Day 5: Body with a Focus on Front-Upper Body and
        Back-Upper Body and Quadriceps vs. Hamstrings
Day 6: Off or Cardio Only
Day 7: Off or Cardio Only

Note*: Start the next week with the lower-body routine and follow the same schedule.*

Sample 3 Day Split with a Push/Pull Focus

Day 1: <u>Push Day</u>: chest, anterior deltoid, triceps,
        quads and calves
Day 2: Off or Cardio Only
Day 3: <u>Pull Day</u>: back, posterior deltoid, biceps, hamstrings
        and abs
Day 4: Off or Cardio Only
Day 5: Repeat Push Day
Day 6: Off or Cardio Only
Day 7: Off or Cardio Only

Note*: Start the next week with the "pull" routine and follow the same schedule.*

Pictures of Some of the Core Exercises

Exercises On the Ball

Ball Squat on Wall

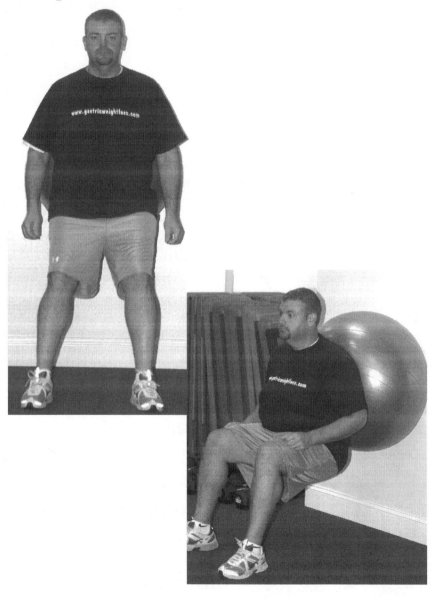

Modified Push-Up

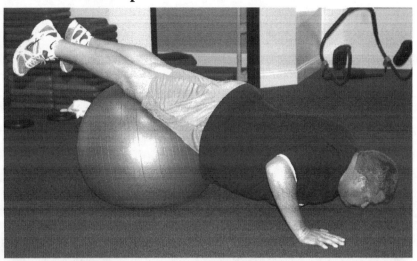

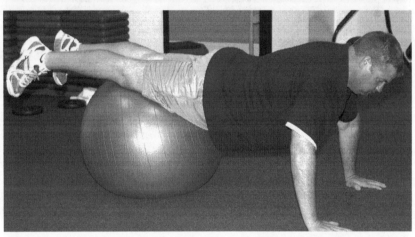

Bent-Over Dumbbell Flies

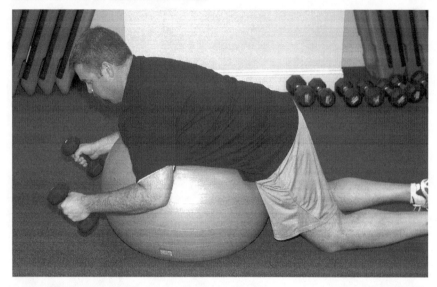

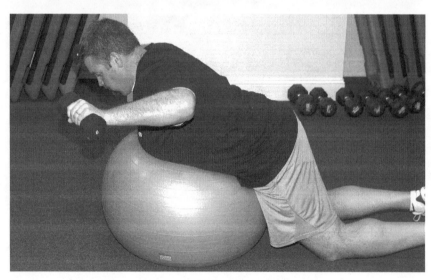

Ball Roll-Back Crunch

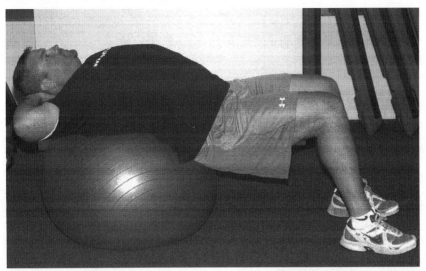

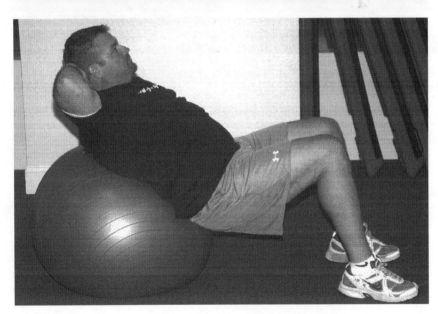

Lower Body Exercises

Free Standing Squat with Dumbbells

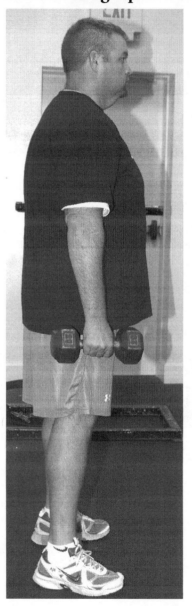
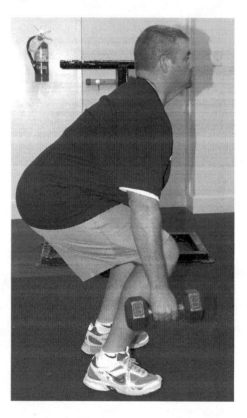

Smith-Machine Squat

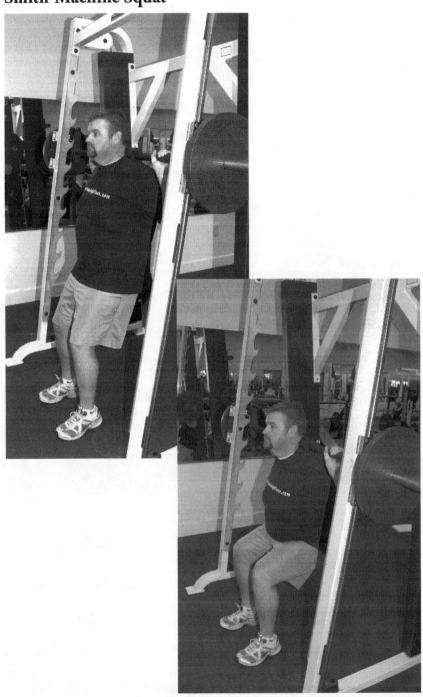

Leg press

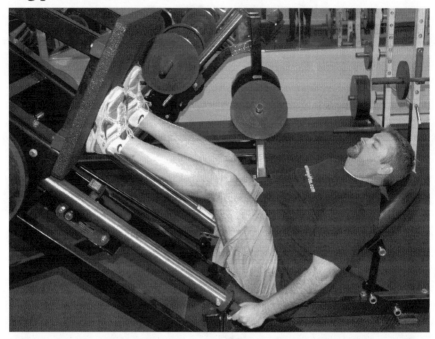

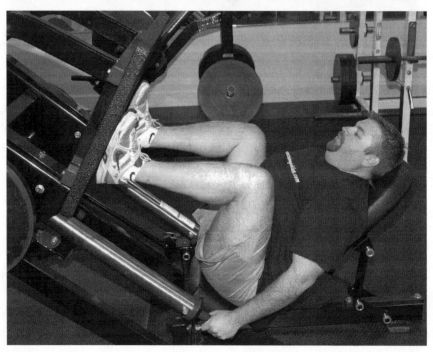

Plie' Dumbbell Squat

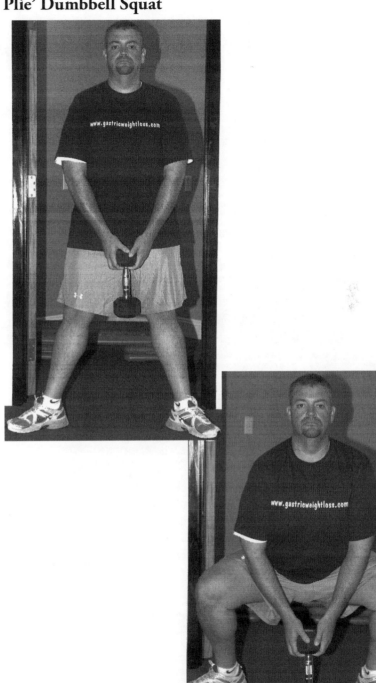

Seated Hamstring Curl

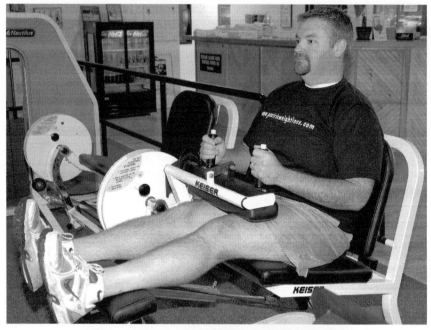

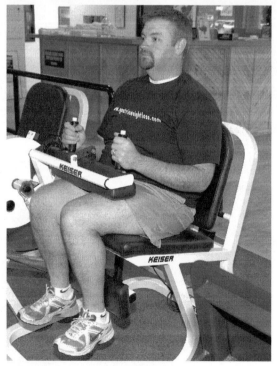

Prone Hamstring Curl

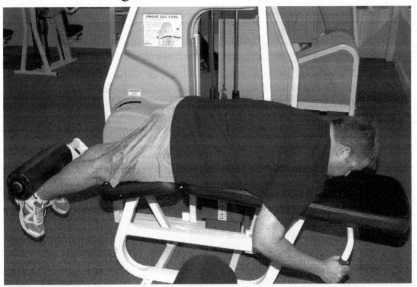

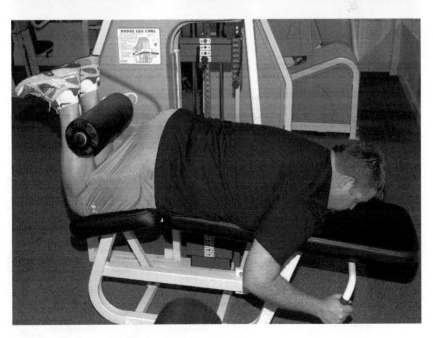

Romanian Dead Lift

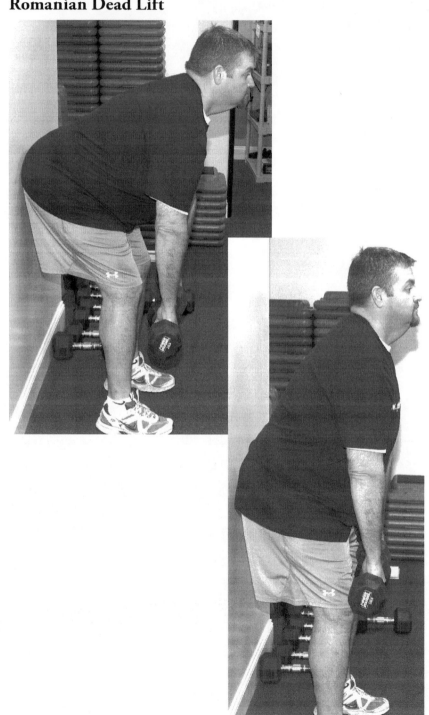

Stationary or Walking Lunges

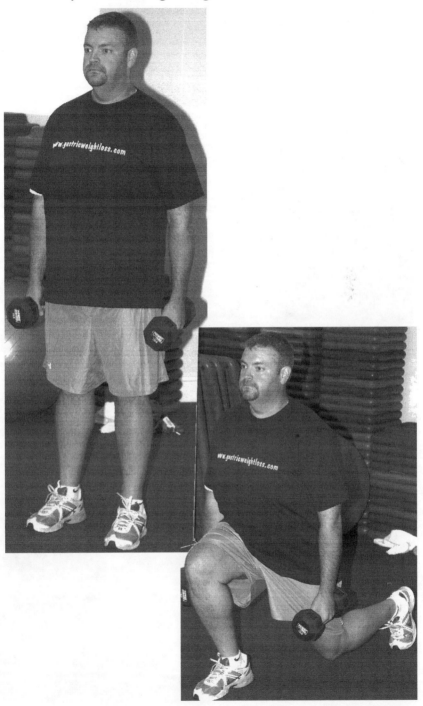

Unilateral Reverse Lung

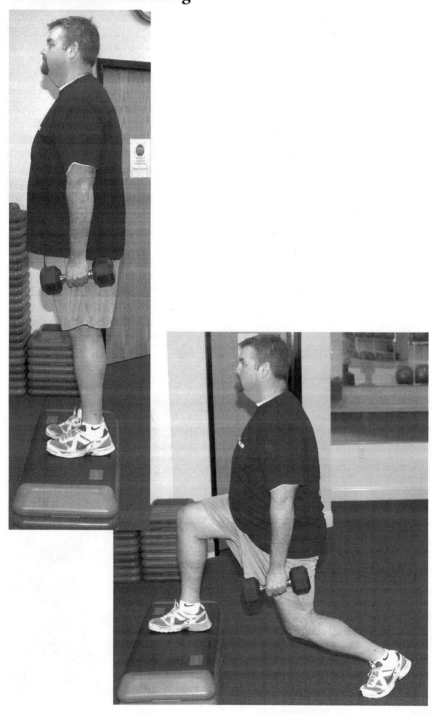

Unilateral Step-Up

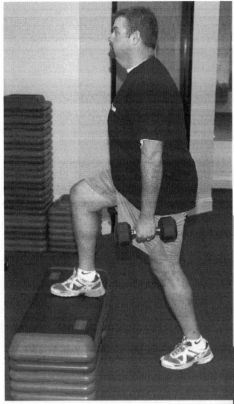

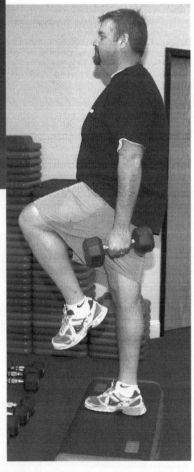

Upper Front-Body Exercises

Seated Chest Press

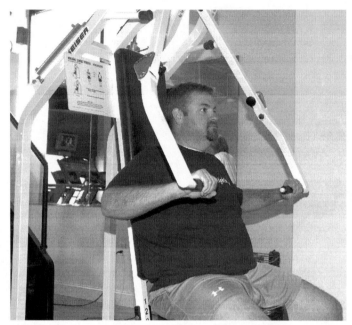

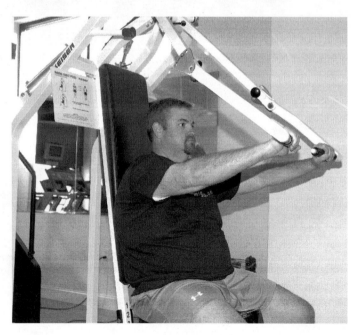

Flat Barbell Bench Press

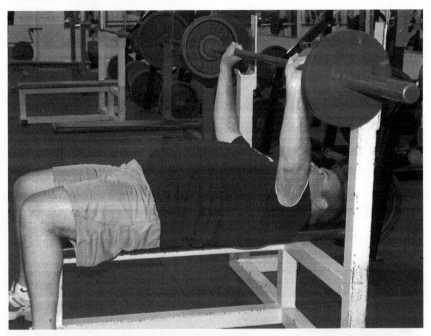

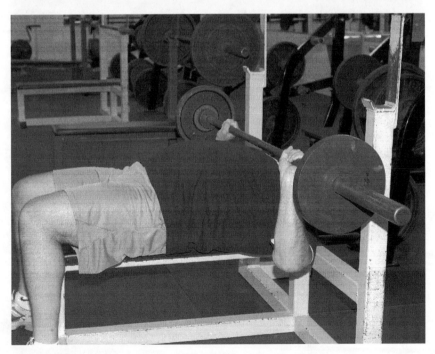

Flat Dumbbell Press (on bench, ball or floor)

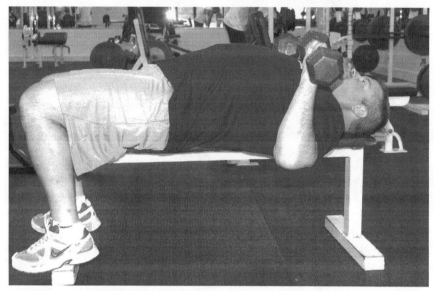

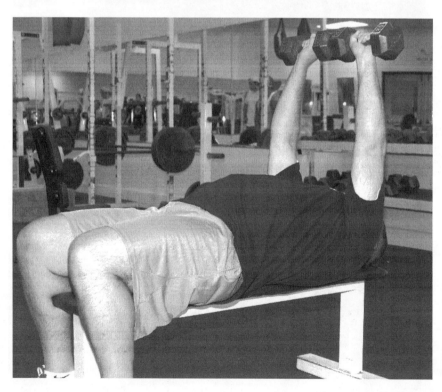

Dumbbell Fly (on bench, ball or floor)

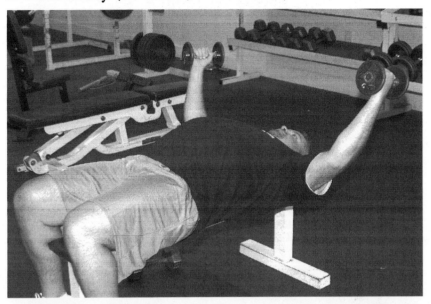

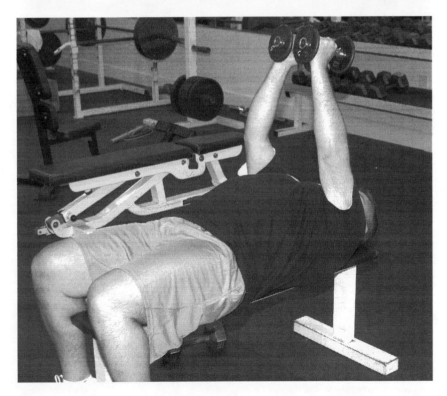

Upper Back-Body Exercises

Stack Row

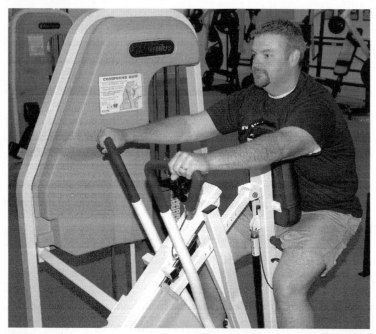

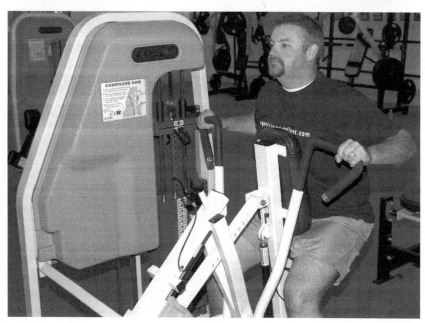

Seated Cable Row

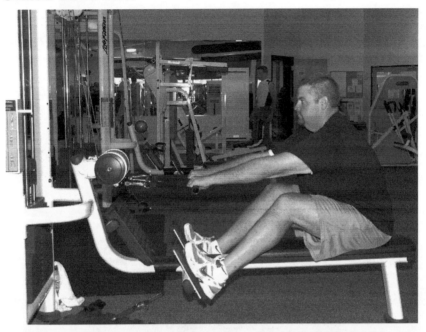

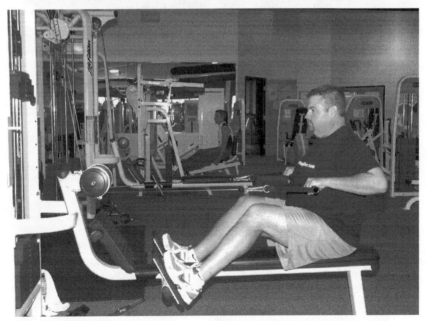

Lat Pull-down

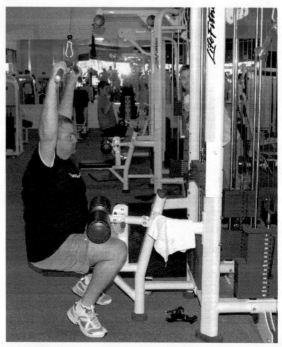

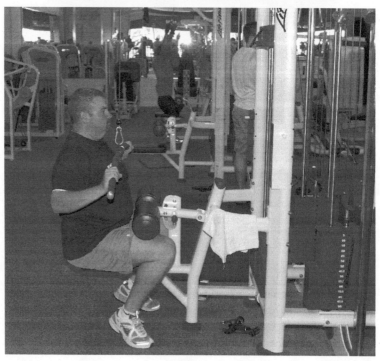

272

Assisted Pull-Up

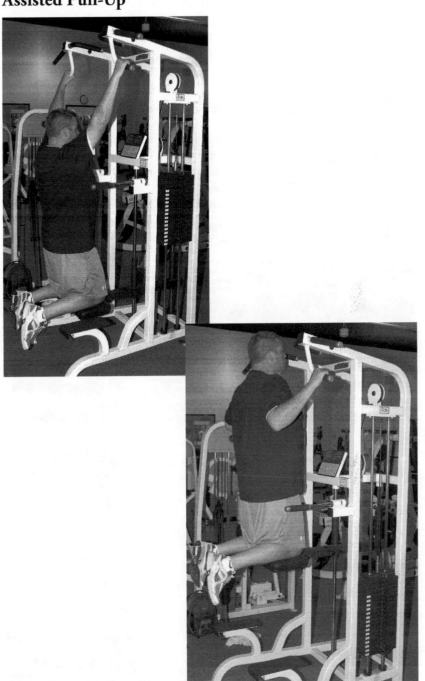

Bent-Over Row (use dumbbells or a barbell)

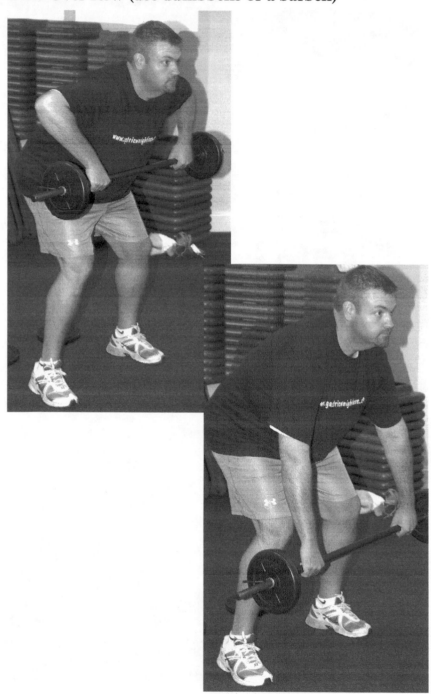

One-Arm Dumbbell Row

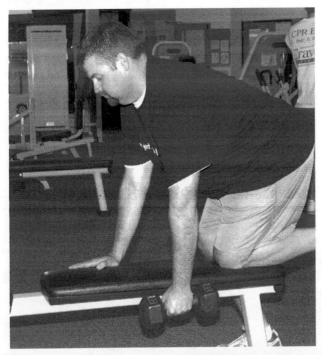

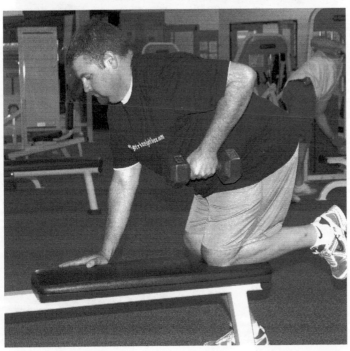

Exercises with Resistance Tubing

Leg Extension (with resistance tubing)

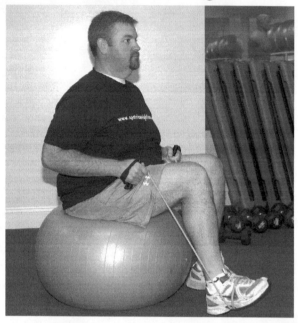

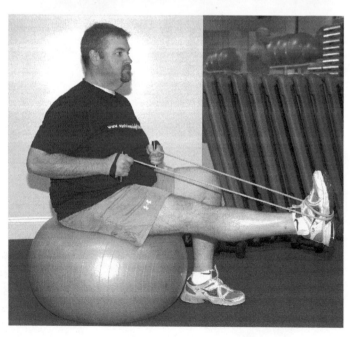

Seated Chest Press (with resistance tubing)

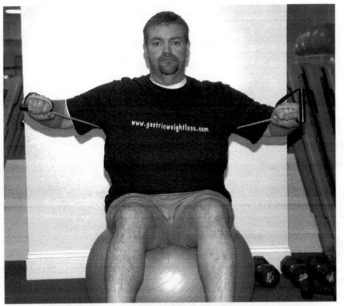

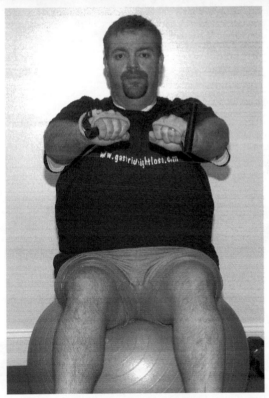

Lat-Pull Down (with resistence tubing)

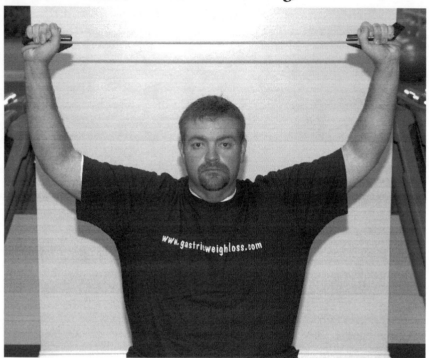

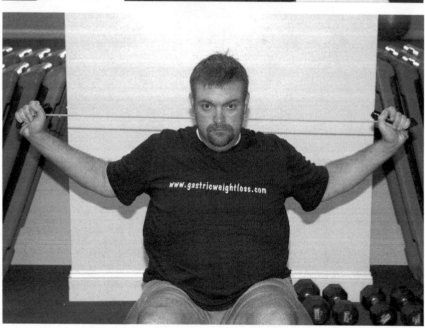

Seated Row (with resistance tubing)

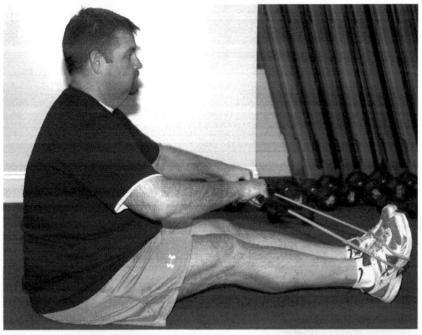

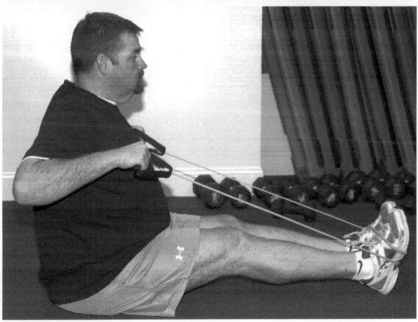

Bicep Curls (with resistance tubing)

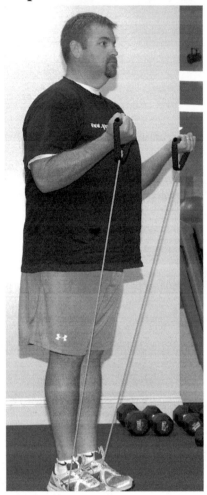

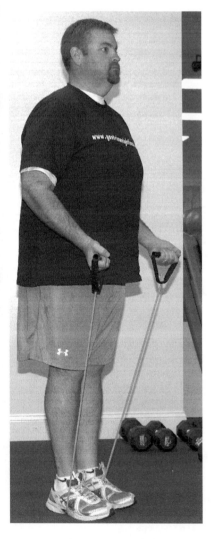

Appendix K

Calculating and Applying your Target Heart Rate and RPE: Rating of Perceived Exertion

> Your target heart rate (THR) helps you maximize the benefits and results of aerobic exercise.

Calculating Your Target Heart Rate
Step One: *Learn to take your pulse.*

To take your pulse, use your index and middle fingers to lightly press the **radial artery** (on the thumb-side of your wrist) or the **carotid artery** (at one side of your neck, just lateral to your Adam's apple.)

Step Two: *Determine your resting heart rate (RHR.)*

Sit or lie down in a comfortable position for several minutes. Find your pulse, begin counting with zero and count each beat for one full minute.

An average RHR is 80 beats per minute (bpm). Your RHR may be *above* 80 bpm if you are not exercising regularly. A RHR *below* 80 bpm is commonly seen in athletes whose hearts are more conditioned and efficient; this means the stronger your heart the less it has to work because it will send more blood and oxygen into circulation per beat. It can be very motivating to take your RHR prior to starting an exercise program and track it's decline as your fitness level improves.

Standard THR charts prescribe the same exercise intensity for all persons of a given age, regardless of whether they are couch potatoes or marathon runners. The **Karvonen formula**, on the other hand, personalizes your exercise intensity to your current fitness level by considering both your age and your RHR.

Step Three: *Calculate your Target Heart Rate (THR.)*
    a)   220 – (Your Age) = X (or your theorized maximum heart rate (MHR)

b) X – (Your RHR) = Y
c) Y x .65% = Z   Y x .85% = Z2
d) Z + (Your RHR) = the low end of your THR range
Z2 + (Your RHR) = the upper end of your THR range

Example: Using a 35 year old with a RHR of 80 bpm
a) 220 –(35 years) = 185X
b) 185X – 80 = 105Y
c) 105Y x .65% = 68.25Z
105Y x .85% = 89.25Z2
d) 68.25Z + 80 = 148.25 (low end of THR)
89.25Z2 + 80 = 169.25 (upper end of THR)
THR range = 148 – 169 bpm

Step Four: Interpreting your Target Heart Rate (THR.)
As demonstrated in the example above, a 35 year old with a RHR of 80 bpm would get the best results from aerobic exercise intensity within a range of 148 to 169 bpm. If the exercise intensity was decreased to 140 bpm or below on a regular basis, a fitness plateau would occur. If the exercise intensity was increased to greater than 169 bpm, the exerciser would be working anaerobically. When working anaerobically you are working without oxygen and will burn glucose as the main source of fuel. Anaerobic exercise reduces both the duration you will be able to sustain the workout and the amount of fat you will burn during exercise.

Note: Your heart rate may be affected by a number of factors such as certain medications, caffeine, stress, illness and a lack of sleep. Monitor regularly for best application.

RPE: Rate of Perceived Exertion

The rate of perceived exertion (RPE) is a subjective way to gauge the intensity of your cardio workouts. Here's what the numbers mean:

RPE 1-2: Very easy; you can converse with no effort.

RPE 3: Easy; you can converse with almost no effort.

RPE 4: Moderately easy; you can carry on a comfortable conversation with little effort. An RPE of 4 or less would be below your THR range.

RPE 5: Moderate work level; conversation requires some effort. This RPE would be equivalent to the low end or approximately 65-70% of your THR range.

RPE 6: Moderately hard; speaking requires more effort. This RPE would be equivalent to the low-middle point or approximately 70-75% of your THR range.

RPE 7: Difficult; conversation requires a lot of effort. This RPE would be equivalent to the middle to upper point or about 75-80% of your THR range.

RPE 8: Very difficult; conversation requires maximum effort. This RPE would be equivalent to the upper end or 80-85% of your THR range.

RPE 9-10: Peak effort; "no talking-zone." This RPE would be considered anaerobic or above your THR range.

Note: RPE can be used in conjunction with or in place of measuring your pulse. Maintain an RPE between 5 and 8 when working aerobically for maximum benefits.

Appendix L

A Bariatic Food Guide Pyramid

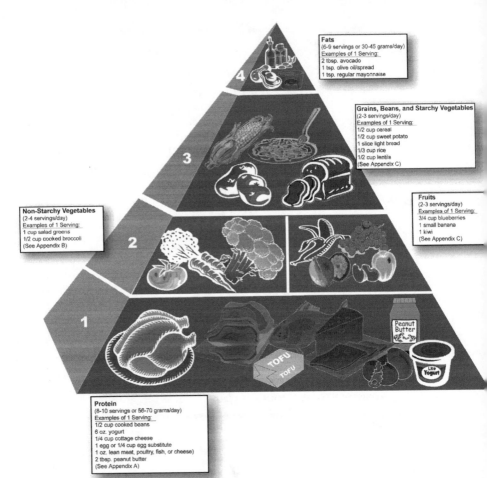

Fats
(6-9 servings or 30-45 grams/day)
Examples of 1 Serving:
2 tbsp. avocado
1 tsp. olive oil/spread
1 tsp. regular mayonnaise

Grains, Beans, and Starchy Vegetables
(2-3 servings/day)
Examples of 1 Serving:
1/2 cup cereal
1/2 cup sweet potato
1 slice light bread
1/3 cup rice
1/2 cup lentils
(See Appendix C)

Fruits
(2-3 servings/day)
Examples of 1 Serving:
3/4 cup blueberries
1 small banana
1 kiwi
(See Appendix C)

Non-Starchy Vegetables
(2-4 servings/day)
Examples of 1 Serving:
1 cup salad greens
1/2 cup cooked broccoli
(See Appendix B)

Protein
(8-10 servings or 56-70 grams/day)
Examples of 1 Serving:
1/2 cup cooked beans
6 oz. yogurt
1/4 cup cottage cheese
1 egg or 1/4 cup egg substitute
1 oz. lean meat, poultry, fish, or cheese)
2 tbsp. peanut butter
(See Appendix A)

1. **Always choose a protein-rich food first.** Ensure a minimum of 21 grams of protein per meal or 60-90 grams of protein per day.
2. **Choose nutrient dense fruits and vegetables second** for good nutrition status.

3. **Choose whole grains** such as whole wheat bread, brown rice and whole grain cereal for good fiber and overall nutrition.
4. **Choose monounsaturated and polyunsaturated fats for good heart health.** Limit intake of white bread, white rice and concentrated sweets.

Appendix M

Anatomy of a Food Label

Nutrition Facts

Serving Size 1 cup (228g)
Servings Per Container 2

(1)

Amount Per Serving

Calories 250	Calories from Fat 110

	% Daily Value*
Total Fat 12g	**18%**
Saturated Fat 3g	**15%**
Trans Fat 0g	
Monounsaturated Fat 5g	
Cholesterol 30mg	**10%**
Sodium 225mg	**20%**
Potassium 700mg	**20%**
Total Carbohydrate 31g	**10%**
Dietary Fiber 5g	**0%**
Sugars 5g	
Protein 8g	
Vitamin A	**4%**
Vitamin C	**2%**
Calcium	**20%**
Iron	**4%**

*Percent daily values are based on a 2,000 calorie diet Your daily Values may be higher or lower depending on your calorie needs.

	Calories	2,000	2,500
Total Fat	Less than	55g	80g
Sat Fat	Less than	20g	25g
Cholestrol	Less than	300mg	300mg
Sodium	Less than	2,400mg	2,400mg
Total Carbohydrate		300g	375mg
Dietary Fiber		25g	30g

(5)
(6)
(2)
(3)
(4)

1. **Check the serving size first**. If you double the serving size you eat, you double the calories, total carbohydrate, protein, fat and other nutrients.

2. **Always count the total grams of carbohydrate**, not just the grams of sugar, to minimize dumping and maximize overall weight loss.

3. **Choose carbohydrate foods that provide a good source of fiber.** Try to include fruit, vegetables, whole-grains and other high-fiber foods at each meal to meet your goal of 25-35 grams of fiber daily.

4. **Know whcich foods are a good source of protein** and be sure to meet you minimum goal for protein at every meal. (see Appendix A)

5. **Choose your fats wisely.** Look for foods low in saturated fat, trans fat and cholesterol to reduce your risk of heart disease. Include monounsaturated and polyunsaturated fats in the diet regularly but limit total fat intake to 30-35 percent of total calories.

6. **Keep an eye on sodium.** Research shows that eating less than 2,400 mg of sodium (about 1 tsp. of salt) per day may reduce the risk of high blood pressure. Most of the sodium we eat comes from processed foods such as canned soups, frozen dinners, crackers, chips, cookies and fast food, not from the salt-shaker. In addition, the DASH studies continue to demonstrate positive effects on blood pressure with regular consumption of foods rich in calcium, potassium, magnesium and fiber. The DASH diet (which stands for dietary approaches to stop hypertension) emphasizes low-fat dairy products, fruit, vegetables and whole grains in combination with a low sodium diet for good blood pressure control. For more information on the DASH diet, visit the NHLBI web site and download the brochure "Following the DASH diet": *www.nhlbi.nih.gov/health/public/heart/ hbp/dash/index.htm*. This brochure provides guidelines on how to follow the DASH diet, including the servings and food groups for the eating plan and the number of servings appropriate to the patient's caloric needs.

About Jerry Wayne

Jerry Wayne is a graduate of Specs Howard School of Broadcasting in Detroit, MI. He is now Program Director and morning show host at Oldies 107.9 in Greenville, NC. He has been in the radio industry for almost two decades and his career has taken him to three different states. He has called North Carolina his home for the past twelve years with his wife Rexanne, a North Carolina native and they're daughter, Anna, who attends North Carolina State University.

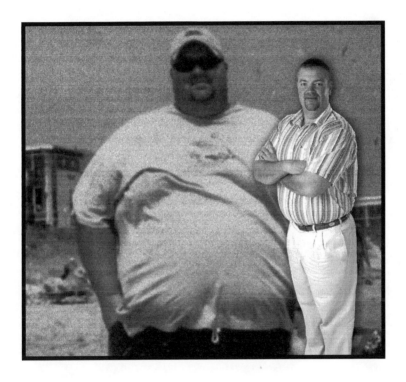

Made in the USA